SWNHS

C20108647

D0544923

3 WM
224
A

Design for Nature in Dementia Care

Library
Knowledge Spa
Royal Cornwall Hospital
Treliske
Truro. TR1 3HD

Bradford Dementia Group Good Practice Guides

Under the editorship of Murna Downs, Chair in Dementia Studies at the University of Bradford, this series constitutes a set of accessible, jargon-free, evidence-based good practice guides for all those involved in the care of people with dementia and their families. The series draws together a range of evidence including the experience of people with dementia and their families, practice wisdom, and research and scholarship to promote quality of life and quality of care.

Bradford Dementia Group offer undergraduate and post graduate degrees in dementia studies and short courses in person-centred care and Dementia Care Mapping, alongside study days in contemporary topics. Information about these can be found on www.bradford.ac.uk/acad/health/dementia.

Design for Nature in Dementia Care

Garuth Chalfont

Jessica Kingsley Publishers
London and Philadelphia

First published in 2008
by Jessica Kingsley Publishers
116 Pentonville Road
London N1 9JB, UK
and
400 Market Street, Suite 400
Philadelphia, PA 19106, USA

www.jkp.com

Copyright © Garuth Chalfont 2008
Front cover photograph copyright © Terry Bruce 2008

All rights reserved. No part of this publication may be reproduced in any material form (including photocopying or storing it in any medium by electronic means and whether or not transiently or incidentally to some other use of this publication) without the written permission of the copyright owner except in accordance with the provisions of the Copyright, Designs and Patents Act 1988 or under the terms of a licence issued by the Copyright Licensing Agency Ltd, Saffron House, 6-10 Kirby Street, London EC1N 8TS. Applications for the copyright owner's written permission to reproduce any part of this publication should be addressed to the publisher.

Warning: The doing of an unauthorised act in relation to a copyright work may result in both a civil claim for damages and criminal prosecution.

Library of Congress Cataloging in Publication Data
A CIP catalog record for this book is available from the Library of Congress

British Library Cataloguing in Publication Data
A CIP catalogue record for this book is available from the British Library

ISBN 978 1 84310 571 8

Printed and bound in Great Britain by
Athenaeum Press, Gateshead, Tyne and Wear

To Mary, Elsie W., Maidie, Winnie and Elsie N.

Contents

Acknowledgements

The opportunity to write this book came as a welcome surprise. First it recognises the level of importance being ascribed to connection to the natural world within the field of dementia care. Second, being a book about design as well as care practice it further recognises that 'environment' is about people and place. Indeed, a successful care environment is just that, a synergy of the two. And, third, walking an interdisciplinary path is a lonely exercise, not arguing any particular professional viewpoint nor having a standard tool kit with which to implement it. To be able to stand at the intersection of care practice and design, and to have the chance to contribute to both, comes as a reward for having been, as one colleague put it years ago, a 'moving target' in terms of professions. It also seems a pivotal point in my 50th year to be culminating in a series of career transitions (music, geography, therapeutic landscape, architecture) at the same time as beginning a new one (design for dementia care), which draws together all these colourful threads into a rich tapestry of insight and optimism.

But perhaps the greatest significance of this book appearing within the Bradford Dementia Group Good Practice Guides series is the opportunity to begin to develop a person-centred approach in which people with dementia are central to the design of places in which they will live out their lives. I was once shocked and puzzled when a famous but disillusioned architect commented that 'housing is lethal'. Although he was speaking in the context of private housing in the community, I now understand what he meant. Too much house design ignores the people it is designed to house. What I hope to do in this book is to bring the voices of people with dementia squarely into the design brief – and not just from the point of managing behaviour, but also from the point of enabling life. As an interloper between professions (including those of family and professional care-giver), my multiple loyalties help me to understand professional borders while at the same time allowing me to stimulate an enthusiasm within professions to extend beyond the very boundaries that tend to define them. For these reasons, and many more, I am grateful to Murna Downs and the Bradford Dementia Group for this opportunity to write about my experiences.

I would like to thank my colleagues and co-investigators for both their direct and indirect contributions to this book. The INDEPENDENT (Investigating Enabling Environments for People with Dementia) project included Andrew Sixsmith, Grant Gibson and Pam Clark from the University of Liverpool; Roger Orpwood and James Chadd from the University of Bath, Institute of Medical Engineering (BIME); and Judith Torrington from the University of Sheffield, School of Architecture. Valued collaborating organisations were SheffCare, Dementia Voice, Northamptonshire County Council and Huntleigh Healthcare. I have also benefited from involvement with older people, staff members, managers and owners of dementia-care facilities, as well as relatives of people with dementia. I am very appreciative of the SheffCare organisation – in particular Anita Bland, Justine DaSilva, the staff and 'ladies' on the ground floor, Rod MacAskill and his team, and Mike Vickers, for their generosity and assistance throughout the research. The INDEPENDENT Project was sponsored by the UK Engineering and Physical Sciences Research Council (EPSRC) as part of its EQUAL (Extended Quality of Life) programme.

My role as researcher on the project afforded me the opportunity to meet and spend a great deal of time with people with dementia and their care-givers, who will be speaking from these pages. Out of this intense and deeply rich experience I was able to produce my doctoral thesis, which informs many sections of the book. I would like to extend my gratitude to Judith Torrington for supervising my PhD, and to Clive Baldwin and Elizabeth Burton for examining and improving it.

I am very grateful to Terje Danielsen, Annelie Sjöström Larsson, Dennis Maciuszek, Torhild Holthe, Sidsel Bjørneby, Carol Edelstein, Claire Moore, Sibylle Heeg, Christer Fällman, Katherine Froggatt, Sue Davies, Helle Wijk, Ad Witlox, Aiko Mori, Takemi Sugiyama, Janet Bell, Jackie Smith and Alex Walker for generously providing time, contacts, materials, floor plans and support. To Judith Torrington, Simon Evans, Linda Evans and Sylvie Silver, and most especially to John Woolham, Clive Baldwin and Mary Marshall, I am indebted for generous gifts of time, energy and willingness, and for editorial scrutiny, peer review, comments, criticism and support.

My main teachers, guides and inspiration have been people with dementia and their families. Most especially I thank them, for their love and acceptance (whoever they might think I am), for their wisdom and humour, for their stories and songs. In this book the words of two particular people with dementia are used with the enthusiastic consent of their son or daughter, in order that their love of life and the joy they both showed in the daily acts of living in harmony with nature should not be silenced by the grave.

Garuth Chalfont
Sheffield, January 2007

Introduction

It is fitting that I am writing this in the dark, cold days of January because, as surely as the bulbs are starting to break the soil, I believe there is a groundswell of interest in the design of dementia-care environments. This is a book about connection with nature. While most of us believe that maintaining such a connection is beneficial for people with dementia, we now have quite a bit of evidence to support this. The difficulty is translating this evidence into practice, which is why this is also a book about design. Nature is everywhere, and the challenge for care practitioners and designers alike is to find creative ways to bring people in contact with it, for the benefits it is known to provide.

Throughout the book, the setting is largely that of residential care, as opposed to care for people still living in their own home. The cultural context is predominantly the UK, Norway and the USA. But many aspects are addressed in a way that makes the practice guidance widely applicable. The words of people with dementia and their care-givers (some in a 'broad Yorkshire' dialect) are interspersed to keep the focus where it belongs and to give fresh insights into the topics discussed. Research evidence is included – dementia-specific where possible – in text boxes you can choose to skip over or dip into.

The book is organised into two parts – Nature Indoors and Nature Outdoors. This is an artificial division (for instance, a doorway is some of each) and is simply a convenient means to organise the information.

- Part 1 contains three chapters: living with nature, nature-based activities and ethical issues concerning nature indoors.

- Part 2 contains four chapters: the natural world, activities outdoors, ethical issues concerning nature outdoors and the summary.

Each chapter ends with a list of suggestions for implementation from three perspectives – the person with dementia, the social environment and the physical environment – and is followed by a brief take-home message.

So what do we mean by 'nature'? Everything on the Earth, except meteorites, came from the Earth. You could therefore argue that nature is everything – including people and everything we have produced. So, even skyscrapers are 'natural'. But most of us tend to think of 'nature' as not man-made but living things, such as trees, grass, clouds, weeds, weather, wildlife, and so on. For the purpose of care practice we can add the stipulation 'beneficial', which rules out typhoid and tarantulas, but which still leaves a wide scope for ways in which nature can be included into daily life for a person in dementia care.

We experience nature in our daily lives in various forms. The spinning of the Earth and its rotation around the sun bring day and night, and the changing of the seasons from winter to summer, depending on where you live around the globe. Weather and climate affect the sun reaching us and our view of the heavens at night, whether starry or overcast. Weather and climate are also experienced directly when the amount of humidity in the air interacts with the temperature to produce mist, fog, clouds, rain, snow and hail. Light interacting with moisture in the air creates rainbows. When air of different temperatures meets, the warmer air rises and the colder air slips underneath. This is the basis for wind and breezes. The climate and the weather interact with landforms and water bodies to create habitat and vegetation upon which animal life depends. Birds need trees to build nests in, for berries and insects to eat, and for protection from weather and predators. The Earth is a marvellously intricate web of interdependencies.

To build care settings while giving no thought to integrating the buildings into the natural interdependent flow of life is a missed opportunity for nourishing the mind, the senses and the spirit. This book deals with the realities in care settings at the moment, but its goal is to increase the desire among practitioners, family care-givers and people with dementia themselves, for more pleasant, stimulating and fulfilling places. Armed with some basic tools and information, the users of the buildings can push forward the design revolution, as the people most directly impacted by the effects of design decisions.

There are clearly some barriers to providing a connection to nature in the built environment, such as windowsill height, building orientation and outdoor access, or in the social environment in terms of policy, risk, health, safety and staffing issues. Other barriers involve a lack of understanding of the benefits of nature for people with dementia and the practicalities of providing such benefits in care settings (see the text box 'The beneficial or therapeutic potential of nature'). Design solutions will be aimed at all three kinds of barrier.

The built environment can provide beneficial connection to nature through room orientation, views, natural light, ventilation that brings in garden fragrances, and independent access to safe and stimulating outdoor areas. But it is up to those in control of the social environment to determine how, when and by whom the room is used, because this can limit access to outdoors, and reduce the quantity and variety of sensory stimulation received. If the building has not been designed to provide such benefits, then care-givers are left to compensate with nature-based activities and outings.

The beneficial or therapeutic potential of nature

Since dementia affects a person's short-term memory, a view of nature and the outdoors can provide useful orientation about the time of day and the season of the year. Previously latent artistic abilities have been known to develop in people with dementia (Gordon 2005), due in part to a progressive reduction in function of the left temporal lobe (Robertson 2000). Therefore, any connection to nature that inspires or nurtures creative self-expression through painting, drawing or gardening is beneficial. A connection to nature has also been shown to enhance verbal expression (Chalfont 2006). The natural world satisfies our need for contemplation, escape, restoration and distraction (Kaplan 1995). Natural environments reduced agitation and aggression in people with late-stage dementia (Whall *et al.* 1997). Since nature stimulates the senses, this can provide multi-sensory therapy for people with dementia. It can also help increase attentiveness to environment, increase appropriate communication, reduce disturbed behaviour and improve staff morale (Baillon, van Diepen and Prettyman 2002; Chung *et al.* 2002).

If a building is designed to provide sensory stimulation, and the social environment is also supportive, further opportunities for interaction with nature exist. For instance, if the physical environment contains safe, nearby and accessible outdoor spaces, and care-givers ensure their routine enjoyable use, opportunities will be created for fresh air, exercise, social engagement and cognitive stimulation. Design for nature in dementia-care environments must therefore incorporate both the design and the use of the building and the landscape. The goal of design is not to simply fill up a person's day with things to do, but to develop environments that actually enrich lives, rather than waste time, including opportunities to simply be still (Bennett 2006).

Part 1 – Nature Indoors

Nature can be brought indoors by providing natural elements or nature-based activities. Chapter 1 discusses ways of living with the natural elements of plants and animals, including sections on houseplants and cut flowers, animals and pets. Chapter 2 discusses nature-based activities such as aromatherapy, horticulture, handicrafts and cooking. Chapter 3 considers some ethical issues arising from nature indoors by presenting some real-life dilemmas.

Chapter 1

Living with Nature

INTRODUCTION

The aim of this chapter is to present practical ways of incorporating nature indoors through the use of houseplants and cut flowers, resident pets and visiting animals. It is divided into two sections, with the first covering the care needs of indoor plants, and touching on some drawbacks to plants in the home, and the use of artificial plants. In the second section, resident and visiting pets are discussed, including a piece of research on the use of an aquarium in a dining room. Animals and pets are increasingly recognised for their benefits to people with dementia, which is evident in the emergence of animal-assisted therapy projects.

HOUSEPLANTS AND CUT FLOWERS

Most of our homes and offices contain an indoor plant of some sort. It may be a spider plant that thrives on neglect, or a cactus we can forget to water. But for some, indoor plants are a private passion, similar to that of keen gardeners who make their plot the envy of the neighbourhood. Indoor plants and cut flowers extend the growing season in colder climates, and can provide colour and fragrance on even the coldest grey day. A bouquet of cut flowers adds a living dimension to a room.

As flowers are often given from one person to another, just the sight of flowers can be meaningful. The occasion on which they were given will determine the emotions experienced by looking at them. For instance, some flowers or colours carry cultural significance through their association with weddings or funerals.

Physiologically, some people are highly allergic to certain plants. Such a complexity of meaning and response in our relationship to plants provides a tool kit for the therapeutic use of plants in dementia care. While further sections address such uses, this section explains how to provide what plants require within the care environment.

Care needs of houseplants

To maintain houseplants in a care home somebody must take responsibility for them. They need the right amount of light, regular watering, and feeding with a liquid fertiliser – needs that are described on the plant tag when it is purchased. Care homes can be warmer and drier than private homes, and this will increase the plant's water needs. Where a plant looks best or 'fits' into a room may not be where it is the happiest. It's therefore important to consider rotating plants around the unit to give them equal opportunity for daylight.

While many houseplants die in care settings from lack of water, many also die from lack of drainage. Plants bought or given to residents as gifts are often sold in a pot with no drainage holes, so their roots rot. Check that a plant is in a pot with holes in the bottom and is sitting on a plant saucer or in a larger decorative pot – both of which allow water to drain out of the soil. Potted plants also need to have their soil replaced at least once a year, as nutrients deplete and crusty minerals build up on the surface of the soil and around the sides of the pot. Upgrading to a larger pot allows the roots room to grow.

If there is an interest in providing plants in a home, but there is nobody willing to care for them over time, you will need to be prepared to periodically replace them. Perennials and bulbs such as chrysanthemums and daffodils, received as seasonal gifts, can be planted outside once they have finished blooming, and will return the following year to beautify the outdoors. This is an activity in which residents can be involved.

There is usually at least one member of staff with green fingers (or 'a green thumb') and an interest in caring for plants. Care home managers should find and encourage this 'green heart' by allowing him or her an hour a week to go round the home and care for plants. Have a back-up person for when the 'green heart' goes on holiday. The following quote is from Doria, a staff member who ran the laundry at one home (all quotes are verbatim):

> And every day since then for about a year I've talked to it, and I've stroked it, and I've called it me little darling, me little sweetheart and I've fed it every week. And look at it now with a flower! And you know I were never more thrilled when that flower came on that, never more thrilled at all. And now you see every time they get a poorly plant now, who gets it? Me, me, I get all poorly plants. I walked in't laundry other day and they said, 'Oh, have you seen that plant that I've gave you, Doria?' And I said, 'Oh yeah, poorly nursery again.' I've got another poorly plant and even that's coming

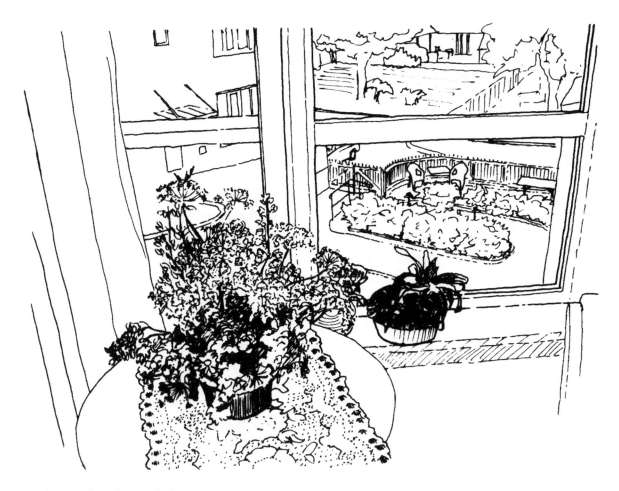

Figure 1.1 Indoor plants and view, Norway

on nice now, that's got some nice little shoots coming on that one. So I get all poorly plants, me. 'Cause they know I'm good to 'em. I talk nice to 'em, yeah. You know you're supposed to talk to plants, don't you?

Residents can also assist in caring for houseplants if encouraged and supported in doing so, which may contribute to their sense of feeling at home by giving them a useful role. Programmes in which residents care for plants as part of the care philosophy are also successful. The Eden Alternative creates a spontaneous environment and opportunities to care for other living things by incorporating animals, plants and children into the culture of a nursing home (Weinstein 1998). Caring for plants can also be a way to enhance family visits by sharing an activity that may have been meaningful in the past.

Other options for plant care are to involve a local volunteer group or to include such care in the routine work contracted by landscape professionals in the home. A local garden centre might be willing to sponsor some plants and/or offer some advice. And finally, in the absence of a 'green heart' you will need to ensure that plant care is routinely done by somebody on the staff as part of good practice, since living plants are silently 'caring' for everyone who visits or lives and works in the home.

There is a myth that live plants can cause problems in a care environment but evidence seems to be saying the opposite. A recent study concluded that plants contribute significantly to the well-being of individuals with dementia (see the text box 'Plants in dementia-care environments').

Plants in dementia-care environments

A survey of 65 nursing staff in ten homes regarding plants in the dementia-care environment concluded that both indoor and outdoor plants were used as tools in the care work. Staff believed that using plants in this way had a beneficial impact on the environment of the homes. Plants created a lush, home-like atmosphere and improved the quality of indoor air, according to the survey respondents. They reported that the contribution of the plants to the psychological and social well-being of the residents was prominent. They observed that plants stimulated residents' senses, created positive emotions, and offered opportunity for rewarding activity. Although the nursing personnel often disapproved of residents moving plants from place to place, picking flowers, or watering them, this study, nonetheless, provided evidence that some professionals in the field of elder-care believe that plants do not cause any major problems in care environments, and can, in fact, contribute significantly to the well-being of individuals with dementia (Rappe and Lindén 2004).

Having said that plants are not a problem, nonetheless one enduring difficulty with having plants in pots in a care setting is that some people with dementia confuse the pots with a commode or urinal. This problem deserves more attention, alongside the difficulties of providing plants (real or plastic) and potpourri that might be eaten by residents. The understandable frustration felt by care staff over such incidents can lead to removal of plants from the unit entirely, depriving the majority of people living, visiting or working in the home, and leading to bland, institutional spaces. The solution involves taking a holistic multi-factored approach, as described below.

This is an area in need of an integrated environmental-design approach that recognises the very specific needs of people with dementia, and the physical possibilities and needs of those who provide daily care. Consider first the person and see what might prompt them to respond in this way. Ensure that as far as possible the needs of the whole person are being met. Acknowledge her attempt to locate the toilet and relieve herself appropriately rather than soil her clothes. The toileting programme in the home and the person's care plan need to be reviewed. May be the person requires glasses?

Consider next the physical environment. Consider whether differently shaped pots that are taller, placed on shelves or perhaps incorporated into the building structure may be more appropriate for the unit. The location, accessibility, signage and door colour of the toilets might also need to be reviewed. Consider the temptation to respond by eliminating plants entirely from the unit, and try to accept instead that some such incidents will occur and plants will therefore need to be replaced periodically.

Real or artificial plants?

In the debate over using real versus artificial plants in care settings, the arguments are strong on both sides. Real plants are alive, they grow, respond to care, improve the air quality and produce oxygen that we can breathe. Plants help alleviate symptoms such as fatigue, hoarse dry throat, cough, and dry or flushed face and also influence feelings of comfort, attraction towards the living space and general well-being (Fjeld *et al.* 1998). Living plants also humanise living space and reduce an institutional feeling. On the other hand, artificial plants, either plastic or silk, do not respond negatively to lack of care, do not need watering, hold their blooms for years, and from across the room (or even up close for people with visual impairment) can pass as real. For care managers, the sight of a dead plant is a problem to be avoided, as it might give an adverse impression to visitors about the level of attention received by residents. Equally, the sight of dusty, faded plastic leaves day after day trying to pass themselves off as real, is equally distasteful to regular visitors to the home.

Artificial plants can also have benefits for a person with dementia. During the author's thesis research (Chalfont 2006) residents perceived artificial plants as real and expressed pleasure at seeing them. There were at least two reasons for this. With memory loss, the person was unaware of how long that blooming iris had actually been in the vase on her windowsill, and so she was able to enjoy it as fresh, each time she noticed it. Also, for a person in her 80s and living in her long-term memories of the past, there is the expectation that flowers indoors must have come from the garden, so obviously they are real (artificial flowers might well have been a luxury in her younger days and were certainly not available very often for working-class people).

Another advantage is that small artificial trees, shrubs or palms can be used in places where a real plant would suffer (for instance, where it is too dark or too warm), thereby adding the look of nearby nature without harming a live plant. Artificial plants must still be dusted or rinsed off from time to time and it's important to replace artificial plants once the colours begin to fade.

Implementation

Person with dementia

- Plants can contribute to a person's well-being (Rappe and Lindén 2004).

- Cut flowers may have special significance and trigger happy or sad memories.

- A person may perceive artificial plants as being real and thus gain enjoyment from them.

- A person may enjoy watering and caring for plants in the home.

- A person with dementia might occasionally relieve himself in a plant pot.

Social environment

- Provide good care to live plants by placing, feeding and watering them correctly.

- See that indoor plants are cared for by a staff person (a 'green heart'), a volunteer, a family care-giver or a professional plants person.

- When possible, involve people with dementia in watering and caring for plants.

- Have a re-potting day each spring, outside once the weather warms up. Use a picnic table or potting bench and organise it so that the residents can help. If a plant is root-bound, trim the roots and/or move it to a larger pot.

- Recycle perennials and bulbs from gift baskets by replanting them outside into the communal areas, so that they will reappear in the spring for everyone to enjoy.

- Avoid use of toxic plants (see Appendix 3). Colourful plants and berries are prone to being eaten, and even non-poisonous plants can make a person sick.

- Remove and replace dead or neglected plants rather than allowing a plant to deteriorate, thus giving the impression that the quality of care given to living things is poor.

- Evaluate the toileting programme if plant pots are being used instead of a toilet.

Physical environment

- Integrate live and artificial plants. Use artificial plants if the look of nature is desired in a space but a live plant would suffer in that spot.

- Read plant tags to determine required temperature and daylight conditions.

- Locate planters appropriately so they are not too hot, too dry or in too much dark.

- Choose shapes, heights or placements for planters such that they will not be mistaken for a toilet. Evaluate the signage, accessibility and visual cues to the actual toilets.

- Check that the plant pots drain when watered to avoid rotting. If necessary, remedy the situation by placing a pot in a saucer or pot liner.

- Choose plants that can tolerate hard treatment and excessive watering, and avoid plants that frequently drop flowers and leaves to avoid extra work (Rappe and Topo 2007).

Message: Provide and care for indoor plants that add a living dimension to the home, as well as artificial plants – which are often perceived by people as being fresh and flowering.

ANIMALS AND PETS

Few of us have lived our lives completely devoid of contact with animals or pets. Whether as a child we had a cat, dog, bird, goldfish, hamster, tortoise or rabbit, or whether there were farm animals nearby where we grew up, contact with animals was often a normal part of life. For older people who grew up in the country, milking a cow or gathering eggs was often a part of daily life. Interactions between people and animals are not only natural but have proven benefits (see text box 'Animal interactions and dementia').

Animal interactions and dementia

A study published in 2002 was designed to test the effect over time of a resident dog on the problem behaviours* of residents in an Alzheimer's special care unit (SCU). Prior studies had demonstrated a significant reduction in agitation behaviours during short-term exposure to a dog. Behaviours were documented one week before and during the four weeks continuing once the dog had been placed on the SCU. Results showed that the people with dementia on the day shift exhibited significantly fewer problem behaviours across the four weeks of the study. The findings of this study support the long-term therapeutic effects of dogs for people with dementia living in Alzheimer's SCUs (McCabe et al. 2002). during the four

([*] Note: the term 'problem behaviours' is used by the researchers, not the author of this book.)

Having to move into a care environment can disrupt people's current connections to pets and animals, leaving the person in what must feel like an artificial, unnatural situation. Separating people from their animals and pets also removes the benefits such contact can provide. During the author's thesis research (Chalfont 2006), people with dementia articulated their enjoyment of pets. For someone like Dorothy, were unsure whether she still took care of her cats.

Dorothy: Don't I look after them now?

GC: I don't know.

Dorothy: No, I don't think I do. Oh, I used to look after everybody and their mother's cat. Didn't I? Every cats on main road. They all come up to my place.

Care-giver: I know. You feed 'em that's why.

Dorothy: I know we did. We fed 'em all. Still, if summats hungry and you've got summat to feed it, 'let it have it', I say. May be wrong.

Maintaining a relationship with animals is not only possible in a care environment, but also potentially therapeutic, and indeed some people in care may be grieving this loss. This section addresses the pleasures and pitfalls of including pets and animals in the lives of people living in dementia care, with sub-sections dealing with pets who both live in and visit the home.

Pets residing in the home

Being allowed to take a beloved pet with us into a care home or nursing home is a rare occurrence. But as care settings evolve into more flexible designs such as extra-care sheltered housing, the possibility that a person with dementia may keep a pet seems to be greater – especially younger people with dementia who are fit enough to care for a pet and walk a dog. They might be less inclined to give up their 'best friend' with whom they have mastered the skill of non-verbal communication. However, with pets there are a number of things to consider.

A dog needs to go outside regularly, which means there needs to be an accessible grassed area that can be quickly and easily reached from the person's room or flat. Depending on the person's frailty, he or she may need shelter at the edge of the building for protection from the elements and also some assistance in terms of picking up after the dog. For people physically still able to walk a dog, there needs to be grassed areas within walking distance, where the dog can have a run and do its business. Developing a routine walking circuit with a dog can be a useful navigational aid if the person develops wayfinding problems. Walking with dogs presents opportunities for both exercise and socialising. In fact, dogs have also been known to bring people with dementia back home when they lose their way. The dog must be well-trained and of suitable size and pace for the person to handle.

For a dog, cat or other pet belonging to a resident to live in a communal home there must first be consent from all the residents and their families, which is often impossible. Therefore, pets in communal environments tend to be owned by the home or a staff member, and often predate the newer residents who give their consent by choosing to move in. Where people have their own flats but share common areas, it must still be agreed by all who would come into contact with the animal. In this case there needs to be an agreed arrangement about who takes over responsibility on days when the person cannot manage the animal, and what happens to the pet once that person can no longer care for it at all.

A more common arrangement is for a pet to live in the home and be a staff person's responsibility. The easiest pets to care for are those that don't need to be walked – such as a cat, bird or fish. A cat will keep mice away, which is useful if seed is being put out on a bird table. However you would also need to put a bell on the cat's collar if it chases birds. It would be important to find a cat that enjoys being touched and picked up. You would also need to check that nobody living or working in the home is allergic to cats or fears or dislikes them, before bringing one into the home. If somebody develops an allergic reaction once the cat begins living there it may have to live in another part of the home.

Fish are an increasingly popular option because they are calming and people enjoy watching them (a reason they are often placed in waiting rooms). Recent research has shown benefits to having an aquarium in dementia-care settings (see text box 'Aquaria and dementia').

Aquaria and dementia

A study published in 2004 examined the effect of having an aquarium in the dining room of a special care unit for people with Alzheimer's disease on food intake, disruptive behaviour and staff morale. The study included 70 people, most with severe dementia, living in three different homes, and used a time-series design with a control group (one with an aquarium and one without). Over a four-week period food intake improved, as did the weight of participants. A significant decrease in disruptive behaviours was noted, as well as an increase in job satisfaction of the staff members (Edwards and Beck 2004).

Visiting animals

In this sub-section we will discuss the two ways in which animals can visit the home – either informally with staff or family care-givers, or in a planned visit such as when PAT (Pet Assisted Therapy) dogs are brought in to visit the residents. In the first situation, a staff member brings her own pet to work. Usually a dog, this pet will engage with residents routinely, providing some of the benefits of a person's own pet (attention, response, familiarity, communication and physical touch) without the responsibilities of walking, feeding or visits to the vet. While not the responsibility of the resident, his or her having access to a pet provides enjoyable activities (whether alone or shared) such as taking a dog for a walk or just outside the building. Alternatively, the dog of a family care-giver can interact with other residents while visiting. A team leader talked about the brother of a resident who visited every day and brought the family dog.

> He brings the dog every day when he comes and they love just to stroke him because he's ever so… He must brush him before he comes in. He's ever so soft. It's quite therapeutic for 'em though, in't it, having animals come in? They love seeing animals. We used to have a budgie. They used to like that. They like it when a pet comes in. The visiting dogs are best.

Animal-assisted therapy involves beneficial interaction between people and animals (dogs, cats or other pets) in hospitals, schools, nursing homes and other settings. Human interaction with dogs is carefully organised for therapeutic effect with a range of service user groups including mental health and dementia. PAT dogs are specially selected for their temperamental suitability and meet residents in the home for a short visit. A more involved programme might also be incorporated into the care plan of the service users. This would involve meeting the dogs and working with them over time to develop a relationship that is beneficial (see text box 'Animal-assisted therapy and dementia').

Animal-assisted therapy and dementia

In a study published in 2006, an animal-assisted therapy scheme was carried out in Essex, UK, working with people with a variety of mental-health problems. Some had not been out of their homes in years. They enjoyed exercising and socialising with the dogs and the people they met. One service user with dementia used to take walks at a very fast pace, accompanied by her spouse. Walking with the therapy dog, she was able to adjust her pace and reduce the stress, not just for herself, but for all accompanying walkers (McColgan 2006). Another study found that use of a therapy dog helped to alleviate the agitation and de-socialisation of people with dementia (Churchill *et al.* 1999).

Implementation

Person with dementia

A person with dementia:

- may have had a long-term relationship with a beloved pet, and then endured separation from this pet as a result of dementia or of entering the care home

- may still believe he has a pet or that he still cares for a pet and worry about it.

Social environment

- For those who do enjoy it, plan for regular contact with pets or animals.

- Consider having a staff person bring his or her own pet to work.

- Consider having animals visit as an activity, such as PAT dogs.

- Encourage family care-givers to bring their pets to visit.

- Consider keeping pets or animals indoors (for example, cat, birds or fish).

- Consider keeping pets or animals outdoors (for example, a rabbit or chickens). (See Chapter 5, p.133.)

- Plan and allow for people to be able to keep their pets for as long as possible.

- Anticipate and resolve the possibly conflicting needs of others in the building.

- Make sure no resident or staff person is afraid, allergic or uncomfortable around an animal.

- Provide help with walking someone's dog, as and when it becomes necessary.

- Decide tentative long-term options for care of the person's pet in the future.

- Plan for progressive assistance with a pet and the eventual complete loss of the person's care-taking ability over time.

- Always consider the animal's welfare (for example, do not overfeed it) as well as the person's.

Physical environment

Provide physical surroundings that support pet ownership such as:

- nearby ground floor access to outside from the dog-owner's room or flat

- fenced outdoor green areas for pets to exercise

- some room where dogs can be dried off before entering the corridor

- a sheltered spot for owners to stand while letting the dog out in the rain.

Message: Connect people with pets and animals to add a familiar, enjoyable, living dimension to daily life, with the potential for friendship, stimulation, pleasure, distraction, reciprocal care-giving and unconditional love.

Chapter 2

Nature-based Activities

INTRODUCTION

In Chapter 1 we explained how indoor plants and pets contribute to a stimulating environment in which people are more likely to engage. For instance, if a fluffy dog bounds into the room, we are likely to react through physical touch. Likewise, if we live in a plant-filled environment we will have psychological and physiological responses that we know to be positive. To complement these efforts to create a stimulating environment, this chapter explains ways of bringing nature indoors through nature-based activities. The chapter has four main sections: nature-based alternative therapies (primarily aromatherapy massage), horticulture, handicrafts and cooking. These are not the only areas in which nature-based activities are possible but these four are included because they have already been used by care practitioners and so others can benefit from their experience. These four also offer different levels of engagement – from receiving stimulation (aromatherapy massage) or marginal participation (such as watching and commenting on the actions of others) to active participation in cooking, horticulture and handicrafts. The success of such activities depends on:

- a person's desire and abilities
- the provision of appropriate space and furnishings
- the presence of natural resources
- the level of active involvement from family and professional care-givers.

NATURE-BASED ALTERNATIVE THERAPIES

Most people are now aware of natural therapies such as homeopathy, chiropractic, reflexology, yoga, acupuncture and meditation. Such complementary or 'alternative' therapies offer symptomatic relief without the potentially harmful side-effects of pharmacological treatments. They are considered 'natural' because they were developed thousands of years ago before modern medicine, and because they adopt a holistic approach to wellness by treating the whole person – their mind, body and spirit.

Alternative therapies use compounds derived from natural, non-artificial ingredients and also offer (through their application method) human contact. They therefore have the potential to provide added benefits to the person with dementia, such as social interaction, communication, emotional comfort and caring touch. One of these alternative therapies in particular, aromatherapy, will be discussed here as it has been found to be of specific benefit to people with dementia.

Aromatherapy massage

For thousands of years, beginning in Egypt and China, people have been practising aromatherapy – the use of pure essential oils extracted from plants with medicinal value for therapeutic purposes. It is a complementary medicine that can be used alongside orthodox medicines to help alleviate anxiety, worry, stress, apathy, sleeplessness and general low spirits. A range of physical benefits can also be achieved, including better circulation, reduced stiffness and an overall improvement in mobility for older people in particular. The fragrance from the oils used heightens the therapeutic value of the massage by stimulating pleasant memories, altering mood and having a generally positive effect (Rigby 1995, p.23). People's personal preferences for particular smells must be considered because certain aromas may have negative connotations for certain people.

The oils are extracted from different parts of plants including the leaves, flowers, bark, roots and stems. Since the oils can be damaged by light they should be stored in coloured glass bottles. Pure essential oils generally keep quite well but are best purchased in small quantities. Once blended in a base oil (for massage purposes) they should be used within six months. An ideal quantity to blend with essential oils and to have available for massage when time and inclination allow is 100 millilitres (3.3 ounces) of a base oil (e.g. sweet almond, grape seed, apricot kernel or sunflower oil). Normal dilution is 2.5 per cent – 15 drops of essential oil to one fluid ounce of carrier oil.

Aromatherapy massage is a common means by which a person can gain benefit from essential oils. Aromatherapy massage is carried out by skilled practitioners, usually for a half hour or more, usually while the person is lying down. During a massage session the therapist will stimulate the blood and lymphatic systems slowly and gently with the palms of the hands using an essential oil, or blend of oils, diluted in a base oil or lotion. As well as having positive health effects, this type of therapeutic approach is particularly relevant to older people because it is gentle and comforting, and can therefore begin to address the lack of caring touch they often experience in later life (Rigby 1995, p.23). The potential to evoke pleasant garden-based memories from the oils of lavender and rosemary, for instance, is an added benefit. Massage can be a loving form of communication for a person limited in his or her ability to respond – for instance, someone who is bed-bound in the advanced stages of dementia. An aromatherapist is skilled in diagnosing a person's specific needs and will select the appropriate essential oils to take the person's mental, physical and spiritual needs into account. The aromatherapist will also know whether the person has any contra-indications to aromatherapy massage (such as a skin disorder or epilepsy).

As well as massage, essential oils can be used in a bath, a burner or by inhalation. However, it is important to note that essential oils should never be added to a bath in their neat form but should be diluted first in a dispersant such as liquid soap. Electric diffusers are now widely available and offer a safer alternative to burners by eliminating the need for a candle. Some oils have calming properties such as camomile, sandalwood and lavender, while others can stimulate, such as bergamot, eucalyptus and rosemary (Rigby 1995, p.27).

There is a common misconception that any type of massage with fragrant lotion is aromatherapy. This is not the case because aromatherapists are trained to use oils in specifically therapeutic ways. However, simple massage of the hand, foot or face can be done impromptu by friends, relatives or staff and still provide a pleasurable and relaxing experience in just a few minutes while the person is seated. Even this form of massage provides pleasant smells and the benefits of caring touch. A team leader, when asked what the residents enjoyed, said:

> Manicures, aromatherapy on their hands, knees, feet. They really enjoyed it. It were right relaxing for 'em, weren't it? Other residents could actually see what they were doing as well and said, 'Can I have mine done next?'

Another member of care staff said:

> Touching. They do like to hold your arm or to hold your hand. They love their fingers doing, don't they?

Even though this massage was not aromatherapy, clearly it was beneficial and enjoyed by those involved.

Aromatherapy and dementia

It is commonly believed that by smelling rosemary oil one's alertness and long-term memory can be improved, while the scent of lavender is relaxing, and both rosemary and lavender can make individuals feel more contented. Therefore, aromatherapy holds promise as an alternative to pharmacological

Aromatherapy and dementia

Smallwood and colleagues showed a measurable sedative effect of aromatherapy massage on dementia (Smallwood *et al.* 2001) and a reduction of behavioural disturbances by as much as 34 per cent. Remington showed consistently reduced verbally agitated behaviours with massage of the hands (Remington 2002), although no treatment group was better than the others for reduced effects over time. In Ballard and colleagues' well-known study (2002) an overall improvement in agitation of 35 per cent by using lemon balm essential oil was shown, with restlessness and shouting being the domains of greatest improvement (Ballard *et al.* 2002). This study supports other evidence that lemon scent improves mental performance, and further justifies scenting areas with lemon scent where mental activities must be conducted under stressful circumstances (for instance, during test-taking). Holmes and colleagues used lavender oil in an aromatherapy stream and showed a modest effect in the treatment of agitated behaviour in patients with severe dementia (Holmes *et al.* 2002).

treatments for disturbed behaviour in people with dementia. For instance, various results have shown that aromatherapy massage reduces agitation (see text box 'Aromatheray and dementia').

The UK voluntary self-regulatory body for the aromatherapy profession is the Aromatherapy Council (AC).

Implementation

Person with dementia

Remember that a person with dementia:

- may have no previous experience with massage and will need to be introduced to it

- may be allergic to certain oils or preparations

- may have cultural preferences, limitations or requirements that affect use of certain oils and forms of treatment

- will have comfort levels that need to be determined and respected – location for the massage, length of time, privacy needs, alone or in a group, sitting or reclining, what parts of the body she allows or prefers, the level of active or passive engagement and social interaction she will want during the process, the level or intensity of visual or auditory stimulation that she finds beneficial. It's important to remember that a person's comfort level can change from day to day or moment to moment.

Social environment

1. Massage by hand with fragrant lotion or oil can be given informally by staff and families.

2. Carry out a risk assessment.

3. Involve and include family care-givers when possible by having blended oils prepared and available for them to use.

4. Introduce a person gradually to the technique. Start with a short informal application to the hands – for instance, applying fragrant hand-lotion or oil for a minute or two while the person is sitting in a chair.

5. Full body massage should be given by a qualified aromatherapist.

Physical environment

- What is suitable will depend on the extent of the massage and the level of privacy required.

  - An informal hand or foot massage can be administered to a person seated or reclining in a comfortable chair.

  - A full body massage requires a bed or massage table with curtains or walls for privacy, space to walk around it and a warm environment.

- Provide a tranquil setting with limited distractions and low-level pleasant stimuli, conducive to relaxation both physically and emotionally.

- Consider using calming music to promote relaxation and relieve stress.

Providing massage in a chair

- Provide two chairs (or a chair and a lower comfortable stool) at an angle to each other so the person giving the massage can easily reach the person receiving it.

- Provide a shelf or small table so that massage oil or other preparations are within easy reach.

Providing massage in a Snoezelen Room or multi-sensory environment

- Visual elements: Lower the overall light levels. Use curtains or blinds to block out visual distractions. Provide illuminations to create both a relaxing and a stimulating atmosphere (coloured lights, a mirror ball, projected images, lava lamp, water tubes with colourful plastic fish moving up and down, strings of brightly coloured or softly glowing lights). Provide accent lighting to focus the person's attention on a focal point such as a plant, a water fountain or a picture.

- Sound elements: Close windows and doors if necessary to eliminate distracting sounds. Use sound-absorbent materials in cushions, carpet, curtains, wall coverings and upholstery. Provide soothing natural sounds such as a water fountain (unless this is likely to make someone need the toilet). Ensure that sounds and music are culturally appropriate. Provide the opportunity for music by offering choices of:

  - acoustic instrumental music (flute, harp, pan pipes, strings, percussion)
  - vocal music (solo or choral arrangements)
  - inspirational music (hymns, ragas, chants, plain song)
  - ambient or atmospheric sounds (rainforest, bird songs, waves, whales).

- As above, provide two chairs (or a chair and a lower comfortable stool) at an angle to each other so the practitioner or care-giver can easily reach the person.

- Provide a shelf or small table so that massage oil or other preparations are within easy reach.

- When using lights and sounds in a multi-sensory room, involve the person in choosing the relaxing or stimulating combination that is most comfortable for them.

Message: Use aromatherapy to provide a person with natural herbal compounds combined with human contact in a way that is both stimulating and therapeutic, and can benefit people with a wide range of abilities and needs.

HORTICULTURE

Part of the word 'horticulture' is the word 'culture' and this denotes both growth and human civilisations, giving us insight into the roots of the word. The development of horticultural skills (from the Latin *hortus* for garden plant, and *cultura*) was what enabled people to stop roaming the Earth in small groups and to start permanent settlements, in which they began growing and harvesting plants, rather than gathering what was readily available. Before the advent of agribusiness, supermarkets and pharmacies, the ability to grow our own food and medicine predicted our survival. Today horticulture is a livelihood for some people, a hobby or passion for others, and, increasingly, the basis for a range of therapeutic approaches to care. There is more scope nowadays for including therapists, such as music or horticultural therapists, into care settings to contribute to the quality of life for residents.

Horticulture can be carried out in a care environment through formal or informal programming of activities or by creating the potential for people to care for plants as part of daily living. Indoors, the actual space available for the activity can range from the small scale (tending plants on a windowsill or arranging flowers in a vase) up to a conservatory, sunroom or atrium. An activity can be accomplished quite minimally in any care setting, depending on the number of participants, and the time and resources available. Horticulture can be carried on year round and can easily accommodate people with limited mobility. This section looks at providing opportunities for horticulture indoors, in terms both of the activities possible and the environments required for them.

Horticulture involves the use of living plant material and can be an occupation that fulfils a person's physical, mental, emotional and spiritual needs – creating fun and enjoyment as well as social and recreational opportunities for people of all ages (Gibson 1996). Horticulture is also therapeutic. Social and Therapeutic Horticulture (STH) is defined as the process by which individuals can develop well-being using plants and horticulture, by active or passive involvement (Growth Point 1999). Horticultural Therapy (HT), on the other hand, is defined as 'the application of horticultural practices and principles in a therapeutic setting to improve the physical, emotional, social, and/or spiritual state of your clients' (Dennis 1994, p.xv). The purpose of a horticultural therapy activity is a therapeutic intervention facilitated by the professional and benefiting the participants, a 'blending of gardening and horticulture science with the therapeutic aspects of life and well-being' (Dennis 1994, p.xv).

A horticultural therapy programme can incorporate indoor and outdoor activities and requires activity space, storage space, growing space, office space for storing records, a budget and professional expertise to carry out the programme. There are also specific programme requirements for indoor space, adaptive tools and equipment, safety precautions and accessibility (Airhart and Airhart 1989). In terms of the physical environment these authors address:

- activity spaces (size, work areas, tables, seating, arrangements and design)

- storage spaces (bulk items, inventory and safety)

- growing spaces (light carts and windows)

- greenhouses (site considerations, work areas, structure, headhouse, benches and management).

The authors present their information within a North-American context and provide two case studies.

Whether working outdoors or indoors, horticultural therapists use a broad range of activities depending on the needs and abilities of the participants and the physical setting (see Chapter 5 on activities outdoors). One of the strengths of this approach is the ability to draw on analogies from nature that can be applied to human life. Gibson describes horticulture as a 'unique treatment medium, entailing the use of living material' and thus 'paralleling human growth and development' (Gibson 1996, p.203). Both HT and STH show positive effect on mood and emotional well-being, self-esteem, intellectual and sensory stimulation, sense of accomplishment, physical and cognitive functioning, range of movement, exercise, socialisation, reduced anxiety and stress, release from depression and pain, outlet for creativity and imagination, and the experience of pleasure and fun (Hewson 2001). Horticultural therapy programmes are increasingly being carried out to involve older people with dementia in horticultural activities in nursing homes and day care centres. The evidence base has been growing steadily, with research showing the benefits of horticultural therapy for people with dementia and specific evidence on the benefits of horticultural therapy indoors for older people with dementia (see text box 'Benefits of HT indoors'.)

Benefits of HT indoors

A study published in 2002 compared participation by people involved in a ten-week dementia-specific horticultural therapy (HT) programme to participation by others in a non-horticultural activity programme. During the observational assessment it was determined that participants engaged in horticultural activities for greater periods of time than in non-horticultural activities. However, the effect on participants of the horticultural and non-horticultural activities was comparable. The authors concluded that horticultural therapy is appropriate for dementia-care programmes serving adults with a wide range of cognitive, physical, and social needs. They recommended that it should be considered as a viable alternative to more typical dementia-care programme activities (Jarrott, Kwack and Relf 2002).

A further study considered whether planting, cooking or craft activities 'engender differential responses' from participants with dementia at a day centre. Individuals were involved in an HT programme over a nine-week period. They experienced success by completing at least one step in any of the three activities, each of which was composed of several steps requiring different levels of ability. Observed benefits included interaction, initiation, concentration and activity completion. Preliminary analysis indicated that the category of HT activities promoted cognitive, psycho-social and physical benefits equally (Jarrot and Gigliotti 2004).

In HT a sequential task can be chosen by the therapist for the participant – a task which has several stages to be completed over time. Successful completion of the task depends on the practitioner prompting or assisting with stages as needed. An activity such as potting up a spring-flowering bulb may include gathering the materials together, preparing the pot and the soil, properly inserting the bulb, watering it in, writing a label, storing it in an appropriate place, clearing up and putting away the tools. Plants should be chosen that:

- are non-poisonous

- are multi-dimensional with uses such as culinary and crafts

- have a distinctive colour, shape and texture

- are easy to propagate and grow

- provide sensory stimulation

- stimulate memory and creativity, and,

- provide meaningful activity.

The following varieties are recommended: dwarf orange tree, scented geranium, lavender, coleus, spider plant, mint, pansy, tradescantia, succulents and African violets (Hewson 2001).

Physical environments

The opportunities within the physical environment for horticulture depend largely on the availability of natural light and on the furnishings. An indoor environment fit for purpose would receive plenty of natural light. The exposure (the direction in which the room faces) and the size and location of the windows and skylights, as well as the geographical location in terms of latitude, largely determine the amount of daylight an indoor area will receive. A room with skylights will receive light most of the day, while a room with a floor-to-ceiling window on one wall will receive direct sunlight to various parts of the room, depending on the exposure, weather and climate. Even a north-facing room on a rainy day will receive some natural light indirectly in the space closest to the window. The spaces in which plants are being grown require more light than the activity space, but the enjoyment of people carrying out the tasks will be greatly enhanced in a sunny room.

A bright, indoor, daylit space with a glass roof (such as an atrium) is ideal for year-round horticultural activities as well as growing plants. While atria are designed into the building from the beginning, conservatories or sun lounges can be added on later. Conservatories (or sun lounges) range in scale from a window alcove to a whole room and are commonly adjacent to a lounge, kitchen or dining room. Such rooms are often too cold in the winter and too hot in the summer. Even though there are some cool-weather flowering plants, such as cyclamen and jasmine, that might enjoy a cool environment, frail older people probably will not. Such rooms must therefore be adapted climatically. Responsive heating and ventilation systems, special glazing, as well as shade devices such as curtains, blinds and screens are recommended (Pollock 2003). On a small scale, an existing window can be replaced with a greenhouse window (a miniature greenhouse that sticks out like a bay window and replaces the existing window), providing shelving space for plants and extending the direction, and therefore the amount, of light that enters the room.

Horticultural activities require appropriate furniture to enable people to accomplish tasks, with tools and materials within reach. Although having a specific activity room for groups to participate in can be useful, other rooms can also be furnished to enable activities. A lounge can have tables and chairs as well as lounge chairs so people are not limited in what they can do by a 'furniture disability'. Families often report there is 'nothing going on' in the home, implying there is a lack of emphasis on providing activities for residents. But most of us will, without thinking, use a room in the way it is furnished and so a lack of activities can be a result of the existing availability and placement of furniture. Simply placing dominoes or puzzles on a dining room table between meals can invite participation in such activities. Is there a writing desk with paper, pencils and envelopes provided? Sylvie Silver of NAPA (the National Association for Providers of Activities for Older People, a charity which sets standards, disseminates knowledge of good practice in activity provision and supports activity providers who work in care settings for older people) points out that when people sit at a table there is the expectation that 'something' will happen. Tables not only afford activities but they also connect people. Even one small table with two chairs at it can make it possible for two people to do something as well as sit.

Activities

Horticultural activities, as opposed to a structured therapy session, can be carried out by care practitioners, volunteers and family care-givers with people with dementia. While such activities are not conducted for the specific purpose of a therapeutic intervention, they are often quite enjoyable and beneficial, and are therefore worth organising and carrying out. Working with plants indoors can provide an opportunity for people to reminisce about their early associations with family members and outdoor nature. Ideal group activities will allow for varying levels of abilities. Two examples are discussed below: a short, spontaneous horticultural activity offered to residents in their seats in a lounge, and a planting and potting-up activity at a table.

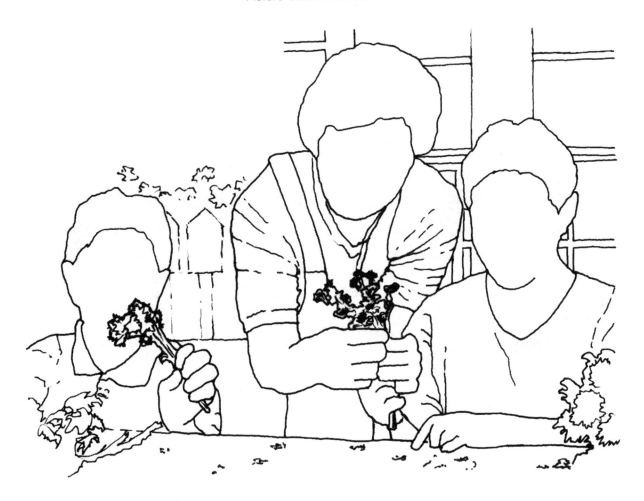

Figure 2.1 Flower arranging, senior centre, Korea

Arranging flowers in a vase is the type of activity that can be done whenever flowers are available, by bringing them to a person in any room. Assume a person can do the tasks before offering to help. Bring the flowers close enough for the individual to see, touch and choose. Do not rush as these moments may revive pleasant associations from long ago. Utilise a tray on the lap or a small table nearby if needed. Removing the lower leaves from the flower stems can be very satisfying for a person, as can arranging the flowers in the vase, especially while having a conversation. Assist with cutting the stems and putting water into the vase only if necessary. Working with a person on his own allows conversation of a personal nature to flow more easily than if the person is with a group.

Conversations can develop because the task at hand and the closeness of a friendly interested person will prompt social interaction. Take the opportunity to have a one-to-one conversation using the activity and the flowers to stimulate discussion. If seated at a table (see Figure 2.1) conversation can develop from the exchanges between people, prompted or encouraged by the care-giver. Clearly people can respond to each other more easily when seated within close proximity, as this facilitates hearing and seeing each other. Both physical arrangements, either individually in a comfortable chair or with a group seated

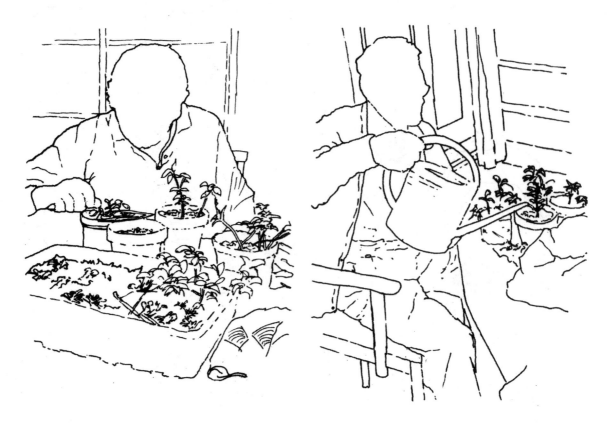

Figure 2.2 Horticultural activities indoors, Norway

at a table, are enjoyable, and also provide opportunities in which to involve a family care-giver. When finished, involve the person in placing the finished vase – maybe on the dining room table, the window ledge or in the person's bedroom.

The next activity requires some preparation. Provide seeds, seedlings, soil and pots for planting seeds and potting up – see Figure 2.2. Seat people around a table so they can participate, watch or converse as they wish. See that everyone who wants to be involved is high enough and close enough to the table. Seat people together who will be able to understand and communicate with each other, paying special attention to seating arrangements for persons with a deaf ear or low vision on one side. Encourage discussion about seeds, trees, growing, farming, or whatever seems culturally relevant. As well as family care-givers, involve volunteers when possible and encourage the conversation to go where it needs to. In horticultural activities provide gloves as a barrier to soil-borne bacteria. Ruth Chaplin, Occupational Therapist with the Young Onset Dementia Service, Manchester, UK offered some of the implementation guidelines listed below.

Implementation

Person with dementia

Remember that the person:

- may have had some positive or negative emotional relationship with plants

- may have physical limitations (reach, grip, dexterity, sight, hearing and balance), which will determine where she is comfortable sitting and what she can do

- may enjoy passive involvement (watching and commenting) but not want to take part

- may have an aversion to getting 'dirty' from soil on the hands

- may try to eat plants or may have physical allergies or reactions to them.

Social environment

- Enlist the skills of a horticultural therapist, volunteer, student or family care-giver.

- Choose a location and time for activities to include those who could most benefit.

- Generate discussion about people's life experiences with plants (flowers and colours they like and why; involvement with older family members in the garden growing up; certain plants or colours that are bad luck; favourite tree and why).

- Use the vase of flowers and the pots of seeds and cuttings as a talking point later in the day to reawaken the memory and the pleasure of the exercises.

- Don't 'over help' a person – a challenge increases the satisfaction of completion.

Physical environment

- Design new homes and indoor spaces with ample natural light, using atria and skylights where possible, or enclosing a courtyard area for year-round use.

- Adapt existing buildings by adding conservatories, glazed additions or greenhouse-type windows. Ensure conservatories are climatically controlled.

- Design and locate activity rooms in the heart of buildings, not in out-of-the-way locations like the end of corridors. Ensure ample natural light.

- Furnish lounges with a mix of tables and chairs as well as lounge furniture.

- Depending on available space, ensure there is at least one table and chair.

Message: Revive horti-'culture' by using live plants indoors for therapeutic and recreational benefit, as well as a tool for prompting memory and social interaction.

HANDICRAFTS

Handicrafts can be carried out throughout the year and can hold special meaning for people, especially through seasonal activities such as feeding the birds or decorating for festive events. Handicrafts can be highly representative of the cultures and especially the landscapes of a people, and therefore they resonate with meaning for people of diverse ethnicity. In this way, nature-based handicrafts can support self-expression and personal identity. For instance, a woman may express affiliations with where she grew up by carrying on family customs and traditions that remind her of home.

Using dried plants

Making things to hang out for the birds and squirrels in winter is done in many countries using dried fruits, nuts or popcorn. Seasonal decorations for indoors are also made and enjoyed, which include the use of pine cones, conkers, acorns, and seed heads from flowers such as the poppy to create wreaths or Christmas tree ornaments. Leaves can be stencilled, drawn around, glued down, painted, used to make a stamp, pressed between paper or hung up. Cloth material, yarn and buttons can enrich the story the handicraft is telling. Dried plants and parts of plants can be used in collages, framed pictures or on greeting cards, incorporating words or messages to create lasting impressions of nature – times of the year, special wild places or outside seasonal events to remember. Herbs harvested and bundled can be hung up to dry adding fragrance to the room, or pieces of plants, seed pods and flower heads can be gathered into sachets and scented for potpourri.

Implementation

The person with dementia

Remember that people with dementia:

- may try to eat the ingredients so ensure you have materials appropriate for that particular person

- may remember certain handicrafts from church or school days

- may have a positive or negative opinion about dried plant materials

- may have physical limitations (reach, grip, dexterity, sight, hearing and balance), which will determine where they are comfortable sitting and what they can do

- may enjoy passive involvement such as watching and commenting only.

Social environment

- Enlist the skills of a family care-giver, volunteer or younger relatives.

- Provide dried flowers, seeds, cones, leaves, plant materials and art supplies.

- Choose location and time of activities to include those who could most benefit.

- Generate discussion about people's life experiences through using the leaves or plant materials (playing conkers, gathering acorns or pine cones, making decorations in school or with their children or grandchildren).

Physical environment

- Provide seating at a table in an activity or dining room, or use a portable table.

- Provide table and chairs at a height so people can reach the items on the table.

- Have a table at the right height for a wheelchair, or consider using a clip-on tray.

- Use a table and chairs outdoors for handicrafts, especially in the autumn when gathered plant materials can be incorporated directly into the making of the crafts.

Message: Use handicrafts to help people express their personal, gender and cultural identity, through seasonal and traditional connections to plants and wildlife.

COOKING

Eating is perhaps the most intimate connection we all have to the natural world because we do not just sense nature, but we consume it and it becomes a part of our bodies. Nature nourishes us and we literally become what we eat. Fruits, vegetables, herbs, grains and spices all come from nature. There are numerous opportunities to connect a person to nature through the growing, harvesting, preparing, washing, cooking, baking, serving and eating of food. What food offers a person with dementia is sensory stimulation from the smell, taste, touch and sight of food (visual appeal, taste and touch all must compensate for the sense of smell which often diminishes for a person with Alzheimer's disease). But food and the way it is consumed is also an expression of a person's cultural identity. People also have very specific likes and dislikes about food all of which comprise their individuality and character. Cooking addresses much more than a person's nutritional needs. People's food habits and cultural choices are a means of maintaining their sense of self, and for this reason food and cooking is an invaluable part of care planning.

Home-grown food

Adequate food and water is essential to well-being. Dehydration is a major cause of ill-health among people with dementia, and a poor diet can result in deficiencies of vitamins C and B, vitamin folate (green leafy vegetables, oranges and other citrus) and iron (Crawley 2006). Research is also suggesting links between healthy eating, including fortified cereals, green leafy vegetables and orange juice, and reduced risk for Alzheimer's disease. In particular, the role of green leafy vegetables is now better understood (see text box below on this subject.)

There is nothing as fresh as food from the garden or windowsill. Having a hand in the growing or even just the harvesting of the very nature that sustains us is satisfying on various levels. Such activities can be accomplished in different ways that cater to our particular environmental resources as well as to a wide range of human abilities. An activity can be planned according to what is available – from an allotment garden to a greenhouse, from a fruit tree to a flower pot and from a window box to a windowsill. Growing foods on site not only provides good food values but also provides the exercise, fresh air and sunshine that are an essential part of going outside to pick or dig, as well as the conversation these activities produce. These sorts of involvements in nature

Alzheimer's and leafy green vegetables

Scientists have considered the decrease in cardiovascular disease among people whose diets are rich in fruits and vegetables, and speculated that this was perhaps due to nutrients such as antioxidants and folate. During a large dietary study of 13,000 women by Kang and colleagues at the Harvard Medical School (Kang, Ascherio and Grodstein 2005), the dietary intakes of fruits and vegetables between 1984 and 1995 were calculated and correlated with performance on cognitive tests a decade later. The increased consumption of fruit and vegetables was not shown to reduce the decline in cognitive scores. However, total vegetable intake was significantly associated with less decline. Women in the highest quintile of cruciferous vegetables declined slower compared with the lowest quintile. Women consuming the most green leafy vegetables also experienced slower decline than women consuming the least amount. What we learn from this is that for those women with the highest consumption of green leafy vegetables and cruciferous vegetables – both high in folate and antioxidants such as carotenoids and vitamin C – their cognitive scores declined less than those women who ate little of these vegetables. This study was able to make a direct link between cognitive scores and eating vegetables, which has obvious implications for the dietary needs of people both with and without dementia.

through home-grown food can entice people into participating, especially if activities are personalised according to the participant's life history (for example tomatoes have a meaningful association for Edith below). Different cultures grow and consume different foods and these differences can be used to help customise the way spaces are used and, thereby, how meaningful such places become. A simple example of this is mint grown by the kitchen door which encourages its use with boiled potatoes. Similarly, in warmer climates it is common to see a grape vine grown overhead where people sit outside. A trellis supports grapes which will be used to make wine to drink while sitting there. These are both examples of vernacular landscapes in which the space is designed according to the ways it will be used.

This conversation about growing your own food occurred with a resident while sitting on a sunny patio.

Edith: As a small child I lived with an aunt and uncle… gardener in his own garden anyway. And he used to grow all his own fruit and veg. That was on Valley Road, further down from here. Um… I think it's nice to grow tomatoes, then you've got your own tomatoes and um, other things like that, to grow food I think's nice, and to grow flowers at the same time. Mmm.

GC: What sort of food would you like to grow?

Edith: Oh, apples and pears (hiccups) oh, excuse me, apples and pears and other fruits, must be lovely, mmm.

GC: How about vegetables? Do you like to grow those?

Edith: Yes. I'd like to, yes, I've never done it. But I'd like to. I've grown the ordinary stuff that you get, you know, just apples and pears. That's going back in time. It goes back in time quite a long way.

Not everyone enjoys productive gardening or is able to participate for various reasons, but a person may still enjoy eating freshly grown produce. Garden landscapes can include a wide range of edible plants (see Appendix 2) that can be designed into the overall planting plan for any site. In this way a meander through the garden can be not just a sensory delight but also provide tasty snacks as well. The beauty of having edible plants in a space designed for people with dementia is that eating plants can be positive and doesn't have to be discouraged.

Living plants give our bodies the highest amount of natural energy possible because once a plant is picked, and certainly if it is cooked, its vital energy dissipates. This is why, ironically, frozen vegetables may contain higher nutritional value than fresh vegetables from the greengrocer, because the freezing process occurs shortly after the picking. The best place to find fresh produce is your local farmer's market because it is usually picked early that same morning.

Cooking can also benefit from using home-grown garnishes that add to the visual appeal of the dish, or flavourings that add to the taste. Nasturtiums and violets are colourful and edible and will add a splash of colour and interest to a meal. Mint can be added to the potato water while cooking to add fragrance to the room and taste to the spuds. Mint in tea is refreshing. Parsley is not only fragrant and looks green and fresh on a plate, but it is also good for digestion if eaten (parsley and other edible plants should be chopped for people who are at risk of choking). Sprigs of rosemary from a bush grown on site can add to the flavour of cooked meats and makes a fragrant garnish and conversation piece on a dinner plate. For more tips on healthy eating and cooking visit: www.healthy living.gov.uk.

The smells of baking

Generally lacking in modern care-giving environments are the sights, sounds and smells of domestic life that are so much a part of our own homes. In particular, the kitchen and the laundry have become institutionalised and

Baking in the Family Kitchen

The Family Kitchen is a concept developed by the author (in 2006) to address the need for family members and residents to interact in a familiar and enjoyable way. The spatial design involved creative re-use of an existing resource – a small underused kitchen in a part of a residential home providing care to ten people with dementia. In its new life as a Family Kitchen, this room enables residents and their family members to spend quality time together engaging in activities such as baking bread, flower arranging or just sitting around the kitchen table, enjoying a private moment over a pot of tea. Such activities engage the person with dementia by a combination of watching and participating, which generates a buzz of easy conversation, while the activity can be the focus, rather than any impairment the resident may have. It takes the pressure off the usual 'question and answer' pattern of a visit. Communication occurs spontaneously as a happy result of doing something meaningful together. The Family Kitchen looks out onto the greenhouse and the gardens – providing a talking point for the residents and their families, and also reinforcing the space as domestic and resonant of normal home life. (Anita Bland, Lead Registered Manager)

Entries from the Family Kitchen daily journal

Thursday, 6 July

Me and my Nan made some bread, just had time to do one loaf – really enjoyed spending some time doing this activity with me Nan, reminded us of when we used to live together. I know me Nan enjoyed doing this as much as I did.

Saturday, 7 October

Made a loaf with her great grandchild, who enjoyed doing jigsaws and spending quality time with her Nan. She always looks forward to visiting her Nan and involving her in all the activities, just like she used to at home.

removed from where people spend their day, along with the sensory stimulation provided by activities such as preparing food and doing the laundry (see Chapter 5 for hanging out the laundry, p.131). For a care environment to provide such stimulation requires practical innovations that begin to undo, or compensate for, the commercialisation of these functions, so that the person living in care can again experience and engage in these domestic activities, and benefit on a physiological, emotional and cultural level.

Clearly health regulations for kitchens and cooking are necessary, as the impact of infections on older people can be devastating. The goal of safety regulations is to provide an environment in which people come to no harm. However, the aim of an enabling environment is to support and promote use of that environment by the person with dementia in the presence of helpful and supportive others – staff or family care-givers in particular. It has been shown in practice that a kitchen can be equipped and used as a normal domestic kitchen by residents with their families, thereby addressing health and safety concerns while also providing a normal living space (see text box 'Baking in the Family Kitchen').

As mentioned earlier, cultural diversity can be celebrated through cooking. The aroma of spices and flavourings of traditional dishes gives a domestic familiarity and is an identifying feature of a person's home. In many non-Western countries cooking is a central activity that may go on most of the day, not just at meal times. Culturally appropriate environments for people with dementia would include the smells of baking and food preparation that they traditionally enjoyed. Culinary involvement could provide an integral sensory experience that extends and defines their cultural identity, as well as potentially strength- ening ties to other people, since meals can serve as the social glue of a community.

Implementation

Person with dementia

- She will know the foods she enjoys or dislikes, and will remember experiences such as blackberry picking or digging for potatoes.

- A person's physical abilities, needs and personal interests will affect whether she has a desire to have central engagement (digging, picking, stirring, kneading, spooning out and tasting) or peripheral engagement (such as smelling the food or watching, listening to and commenting on the actions of others).

- Everyone will have cultural preferences and traditions concerning foods, spices, methods of cooking and serving food and drinks.

- People may also be aware of occasions and times of the day and the year when certain dishes are appropriate or expected.

- The person may have participated in a home life where cooking permeated the day.

Social environment

- Provide a kitchen that residents and families are able to use together.

- Prepare risk assessments for kitchen areas where residents participate.

- Integrate home-grown or home-made food into the menu.

- Encourage family care-givers and residents to prepare and eat food in the home.

- Promote the planting of fruit and vegetables on site and close to the unit.

- Encourage gardening involvement from care-givers.

- Know your edible plants and promote their planting and use indoors and out.

- Engage the person in the outdoors through the use of edible landscaping.

- Incorporate leafy green vegetables into the diet of residents.

- If a person tends to eat indoor plants encourage this by providing edible plants in areas he routinely accesses, thereby reframing a negative behaviour.

- Be aware of the cultural needs and traditions of people and use these to further their involvement and interaction with others through cooking and eating.

- Add edible flowers to the dinner plate to stimulate health and discussion.

- Encourage discussion on the topic of cooking and using plants from the garden.

- Support regular cooking in the home for the person's active or passive enjoyment.

- Ensure the diet provided is culturally appropriate for people living in the home, including the availability and use of herbs, spices and flavourings they use and identify with.

Physical environment

- Provide access to and use of a kitchen space with table and chairs, sink, fridge, breadmaker, toaster, kettle, utensils, bowls, tableware, aprons and tea towels.

- Provide a space such as a family kitchen within 'aroma distance' of seating areas, so the smell of baking bread or percolating coffee can be enjoyed.

- Consider designing a large family-style eat-in kitchen in the same room as the dining area. People can then spend their day in this room, where they can be involved directly or peripherally with food preparation, relax in comfortable chairs on the periphery of the action, play games at a games table, enjoy a view into the garden, take a short walk to the greenhouse, and where there is always something to do – something being prepared and cooked, or a meal being cleared away, washed and tidied up.

- Build a raised area of edible vegetables and herbs within easy reach of the person.

- Include edible landscape plants into the overall planting plan, considering the abilities and needs of individuals using the building, and whether they will have independent or supported access to the landscape.

Message: Bring back the domestic pleasures of harvesting, preparing and consuming food and drink, to reawaken the social, sensual and cultural experiences they provide.

Chapter 3

Ethical Issues Concerning Nature Indoors

INTRODUCTION

When we ask ourselves, 'Am I doing the right thing?' that is the clue that we are dealing with an ethical dilemma. On a practical level, dementia care often involves ethical issues because we are often making decisions for another person – in particular, constraints and choices are often imposed on older people with dementia (Tyrell 2007). As a result 'their rights and freedom to decide are often limited', and since the older person is 'at risk' it is 'in the interest of that person, or in the interest of others, to restrict his liberty or freedom' (Tyrell 2007, pp.176–7). For reviews of the literature on the ethics of decision-making by families of people with dementia see Baldwin *et al.* 2002 and Hughes *et al.* 2002. Ethical practice is 'about asking questions that shed light on various dilemmas that can arise in considering what is appropriate care for people with dementia'(ASTRID 2000, p.40).

Consent is central to the ethics of dementia because it raises the question of whether or not a person with dementia can actually give consent. Does that person understand what they are consenting to, and once they have given consent do they remember having done it? Furthermore, do they have the information required, are they able to make a decision and do they understand the implications of that decision? To address the issue of consent, the ASTRID (A Social and Technological Response to meeting the needs of Individuals with Dementia and their carers) project puts forward these four suggestions:

- Ask the person with dementia herself or himself.

- Communication includes not only language, but non-verbal communication.

- Relatives may need to be involved and conflicts of interest can occur.

- Use ethical protocols to safeguard the interests of people who cannot consent.

Consent involves the issue of mental capacity. In this area Scotland enacted the Adults with Incapacity Act 2000 and in England and Wales the Mental Capacity Act of 2005 provides a statutory framework to empower and protect vulnerable people who are not able to make their own decisions. Key principles of the 2005 Act involve a presumption of capacity, the right to be supported in decision-making, best interests and least restrictive intervention. It further states that a lack of capacity cannot be established merely by reference to a condition – for instance, dementia.

Dementia care also involves ethical issues because we are concerned with the issue of personhood (Gilleard 1984), a concept central to good practice. Kitwood was later to define this as '…a standing or status that is bestowed upon one human being by others, in the context of relationship and social being' (Kitwood 1997, p.8). Gilleard (1984) mentioned dementia specifically as 'the loss of the person' (p.18) and the 'fading of self' (p.10). Ethics is therefore relevant to dementia practice philosophically in asking whether or not the person with dementia remains, in spite of the illness.

Others have also said that 'the threatened loss of self does not appear to be linked to the "progress" of the disease but rather to the related behaviour of significant others' (Bond and Corner 2001, p.104). This relationship view of personhood could lead into various ethical frameworks, including personalist ethics (Schotsmans 1999) or the ethics of care (Tronto 1998).

Recognising that ethics in dementia care are as 'messy' as life itself, we do what we hope will be in the best interest of the person with dementia. However, a good starting point when ethical issues arise is to consider the following four widely known bio-ethical principles that help illuminate the conflicts:

- Autonomy (the person has the opportunity to give or withhold consent, to take risks, to choose what she wants to do)

- Beneficence (doing one's best, putting the person's well-being first)

- Non-maleficence (not harming the person)

- Justice (treating the person in the same way as other people, ensuring that he or she gets a fair share).

'The principle of safeguarding the rights and quality of life of the individual and their family is central to ethical practice' (Christie 2007, p.199).

Risk is another significant aspect of ethics from two perspectives. First, to what extent do our care practices put a person at risk, and, second, to what extent do our care practices diminish quality of life by being overly risk-averse? Exactly what is at risk, and are we making attempts to prevent harm that are *of equal magnitude* to the scale of harm we hope to prevent? Simply put, 'What is the worst that could happen?' We must answer this and then take necessary precautions for the safety and security of those people in our care. Also, we must ask, 'What is the best that could happen?' In other words, what opportunity is there to increase a person's overall enjoyment of life – or even to create one sparkling moment? From this we arrive at what is reasonable. Design of newer homes seems to be addressing only the first question. However, life is a risky business, and it seems to the author that it is unethical to prevent someone from taking reasonable risks *with himself or herself* as part of daily life, if we are using that person's dementia as the justification for doing so.

ETHICAL DILEMMAS

In this section we address some of the ethical issues raised by nature indoors by applying ethical principles (ASTRID 2000) and by addressing consent, safety, risk and opportunity, mental health and human rights where appropriate. All the dilemmas given below are taken from real life and raise certain questions. The decisions that were made are not necessarily advocated as the 'right' thing to do, nor are they the only ones, but they do provide examples of how to reach solutions, which we hope will be ethical ones. We also provide design solutions for either the physical or the social environment where possible.

Eating houseplants and the use of living versus fake plants

We want to have living plants and bowls of potpourri in the home but one resident tends to eat them.

The dilemma here is that all the residents, staff and visitors are denied potential well-being from the benefits of indoor plants and fragrant potpourri, in order that one resident is spared potential ill-being from eating them. Here it was decided to play it safe and put in silk flowers, from which residents gain some emotional if not physiological benefit, because they think they are real anyway. When a resident comments on the lovely fresh flowers, we choose not to make her aware that the flowers are fake, so as not to diminish her enjoyment. It is perhaps more memory loss and diminished eyesight than dementia that enables a person to think flowers are fresh that have been 'blooming' for two years. We are not intentionally fooling people but neither are we creating authentic environments. Is it ethical to let people think plants are real when they are fake? This is a situation to which we might ask three simple questions: Is it true? Is it necessary? And is it kind? These three questions are not a protocol but simply a way of clarifying some of the issues involved. If telling the truth is unnecessary and the person will pay an emotional cost, who benefits from telling it? Not all solutions are kind and necessary, even if they are true. One design solution might be to install a shelf high up where plants can still be watered, seen and enjoyed, and to purchase a long-handled watering can to do so.

Gaining consent for aromatherapy

We know a person with advanced dementia who will benefit from aromatherapy massage, but the family members when consulted did not support the idea.

> From our perspective we know that the person could benefit, especially since the person's dementia is advanced. Here we would have to ensure non-maleficence by making sure the person has no allergies to the massage oil and there is nothing in the care plan or medical history prohibiting treatment. If the principle of autonomy is applied, the person with dementia is allowed the opportunity to take risks and to choose what he wants. From the perspective of the family care-giver, she might be unfamiliar with the process or the benefits of aromatherapy.
>
> Solutions might include offering the family care-giver a massage herself, so she has some subjective experience to inform her decision, or invite her along to a session when other residents are enjoying aromatherapy, and the aromatherapist is on hand and can speak with her or show her a research article. To ensure justice (treating the person the same way as other residents in getting a fair share) one could accept 'no', educate and ask again at a later time. Consent is specific, so a person may have the capacity to consent at one time, but not at another. Importantly, it cannot be assumed that the person is incapable of giving consent, according to the Mental Capacity Act 2005. Appropriate help in making a decision could involve non-verbal communication such as gesture and body language. For instance, if the person allows you to hold his hand and massage it, he is assenting (as opposed to consenting) to the interaction, thus enabling him to demonstrate capacity.

Informing about the death of a pet

A resident's budgie dies because she feeds it left-over dinners such as meat and potato pie. Do we tell her, or do we run out and buy another budgie?

> From this resident's perspective the bird is a beloved companion so one could argue that saving her the grief of losing it is beneficent, and covering up the death is non-maleficent and prevents a potentially hard blow to her mental health. If we tell her the bird died, she may not remember by the next day, and we will need to repeat the sad news, until she forgets about the bird. Repeatedly telling a person bad news may not be necessary and is not kind. If we explain

how the bird died and urge her not to feed it leftovers, she may forget our advice. To replace the bird we are willingly subjecting it to meat and potato pie, and its eventual demise, which is unethical on other grounds. If we put a sign on the cage saying 'People food makes me sick', and supply proper bird food, this will not match the resident's reality, which is 'I've been feeding him pie for years and it hasn't hurt him yet.' Given this dilemma, the staff in this situation replaced the bird (more than once!) because they felt the pleasure and companionship it brought the person was the ultimate good. But in reality, even that solution was unethical as it did not ensure the welfare of the birds.

Food handling by residents

We want to involve a person in food preparation at meal times, but regulations forbid the eating of food that is not prepared in the central kitchen.

Participation in familiar domestic activities such as snapping beans or peeling potatoes is a beneficial contribution to personhood – as is even being able to butter a piece of toast. On the principle of justice, this treats the person with dementia the same way as other people, and it helps him or her maintain some autonomy.

From the health and safety perspective, food handling by residents is risky both in their use of kitchen tools and in the food being safe enough to eat. If we ask ourselves what is the worst that could happen here, we realise that the risk of sickness and infection could have a devastating effect on the whole home.

From the person's perspective, to help in meal preparation normalises the place, makes it feel more like a real home and provides the person with a meaningful and useful role. It also stimulates reminiscence, as the person grew and ate food from the garden earlier in life, recalling with pride the victory gardens during the war, sharing food with others and being resourceful during a time of shortage. Someone suggested having two sets of vegetables so some can be prepared and thrown away, but wasting food is also unethical.

Solutions here include the following.

- Allow the person to be involved in baking and bread-making that does not include meat, fruit or vegetables.

- Educate the inspectorate with research findings on the benefits of involving people with dementia in cooking and food preparation, and working together to establish best practice guidelines for safe food-handling by residents.

- Use consistent best practice in terms of hand-washing.

- With the new emphasis on healthy eating and nutrition, fruit is expected to be left out for residents. Through a risk assessment, determine how and to what extent a person with dementia can assist with this.

- Find, read disseminate articles on the topic to generate discussion and ideas.

- On a case-by-case basis, determine the needs, abilities and associated risks for individuals, and design person-centred solutions, like scrubbing potatoes, snapping peas or buttering their own toast at the breakfast table.

Keeping a pet and moving into care

A woman refuses to move into a care home because she will have to give up her cat.

Many homes have a 'no pet' policy for innumerable practical reasons. However, their policy does not respect this person's autonomy as she clearly identifies what is important to her. The question arises as to whether the person is harmed by giving up her cat – is the policy non-maleficent? The therapeutic value of pets to people with dementia is becoming more widely recognised, as well as the importance of emotional attachments. But do we have any research on the negative effects of giving up a pet? How impractical would it be for people in communal living environments to be able to have pets? What design would be needed to facilitate that? Would this person be able to function in an extra-care sheltered scheme where she might be able to keep the pet? Are there any schemes in her area and is she eligible? Solutions include:

- a family member adopting the pet and regularly bringing it on visits to the home

- the person having regular visits to the family home and enjoying the pet there

- pet-assisted therapy being taken on board, with 'PAT cats' regularly visiting

- the woman and her cat moving into an extra-care sheltered scheme.

Reaction to pets in the home

A home adopts a cat as a pet, but later a resident has an allergic reaction.

The residents had been asked beforehand but nobody had objected. However, a few days after the cat moved in, one resident developed a respiratory problem, indicative of an allergy to cats. The other residents either like the new cat (because they benefit from it emotionally, and encourage it to come into their rooms and jump on their bed) or they ignore it. The allergic resident becomes increasingly unwell, especially since the cat now comes in and jumps on her bed. This resident, who is a stroke victim, cannot easily shoo the cat away and she needs to keep her bedroom door open, so she has visual access to care staff in the corridor when she needs assistance.

One solution is to arrange for the cat to live in another part of the home and to be brought to visit individual residents, who can also go to visit it in the other part of the home. This is explained in a resident's family meeting as a 'win–win' situation, since no one is unfairly disadvantaged. This could also work if the home had a dog and one resident was frightened by it.

Fresh air is a fire hazard

Fire regulations state that bedroom doors and windows must be closed at night, but Mr B cannot go to sleep with his door and window closed.

From Mr B's perspective, this is about his autonomy to be able to choose what he wants to do. He has been told this is his 'home' and has been encouraged to remain independent and make choices, so this rule seems illogical to him. It's important that his perspective is heard and if possible the cause of the need uncovered. It may be about access to fresh air or freedom of movement. There could also be unresolved fears or unvoiced personal discomforts. Was Mr B ever in a bomb shelter? Is he too hot at night and does he need a lighter bed cover? Is he getting enough oxygen into his lungs when he sleeps? Does the home smell? From the regulatory perspective, the safety issue is obvious – the regulation is intended to safeguard lives. But does Mr B have enough information? Has somebody explained who needs the windows closed and why? Nonetheless, even if the issue is explained to him, he may not understand the consequences of his needs on the safety of others.

Access to fresh air is physically and psychologically beneficial, and therefore potentially a human rights issue, but in reality, communal living does infringe on the human rights of some if it is to operate for the common good of all. What is the worst that could happen? If a fire door is propped open the consequences are unbearably horrific. What is the best that can happen? One person sleeps well. If, as mentioned above, we are making attempts to prevent harm that is of equal magnitude to the scale of harm we hope to prevent, then we must abide by the fire regulations to the fullest extent possible. This does not, however, eliminate the potential that through careful design an ethical solution for this individual can be reached, while simultaneously safeguarding the lives of everyone. Design is truly beautiful when it achieves both. However, the question of design raises the issue of cost. An automatic closer could be installed on the bedroom door, which will prop the door open but close it automatically in the event of fire. Clearly this device will have an initial cost. But spending money here to prevent the door from being wrongly propped open is not only person-centred, but could also avert a tragedy. Here, finding a design solution is a cheap alternative when considering the potential human cost.

SUMMARY

This chapter has looked briefly at some of the ethical issues raised by nature indoors. Providing access to nature may not at first glance seem to carry the same weight of ethical decisions regarding end-of-life care, medication, technology or financial matters. However, the same issues arise in this area – such as consent, safety, risk, opportunity. Decisions that impact a person's relationship with a beloved pet, for instance, touch on deep emotional and spiritual matters and are therefore not to be dismissed lightly. We must therefore weigh up risks and opportunities and apply design solutions creatively, while remembering that dilemmas rarely have perfect solutions. When we clearly know what to do in a situation and there is no debate or concern for doing the right thing, there is no ethical issue. Mahatma Gandhi once said that, 'honest disagreement is often a good sign of progress'. How we resolve disagreement ethically relies not only on the quality of our care-giving, but also on the role that design plays by increasing the options from which we can choose.

Part 2 – Nature Outdoors

In this part of this book we consider opportunities to enhance a person's connection to nature in one of two ways – either by integrating it into the design of the building, or by doing activities outside. Chapter 4 contains sections on looking out and watching, integrating indoors and outdoors at the building edge and supporting wildlife. Chapter 5 is the most extensive and contains six sections of outdoor activities, ranging from simply going outside through to taking a trip out. Chapter 6 rounds out Part 2 with ethical issues about nature outdoors and Chapter 7 contains seven key points, sections on design research and ecological sustainability, and some concluding comments.

Part 2 – Native Outdoors

Chapter 4

The Natural World

INTRODUCTION

The way in which people experience the outside world can be enhanced through design of their built and social environment, and in this chapter we look at three ways in which aspects of a building enable nature to penetrate it. First, we look at how an activity as simple as looking out of the window and watching the world go by depends on variables such as what the view from the window contains, where the room is located in the building, where the building is located on the land, where in the building a person spends time and how much access he or she has to assistive technology.

A second way of enhancing the experience of outdoor nature for a person indoors depends on how well the building integrates indoors and outdoors at the building 'edge'. The exterior wall, instead of being a barrier between indoors and outdoors, can be made more permeable by attention to the height and placement of windows and furniture, the location and design of transitional spaces and the provision of cloisters and covered walkways.

A third way in which a person's experience of outdoor nature can be improved is to support wildlife through maintaining the health, diversity and nearness of habitats and ecosystems, and the presence of wildlife in urban environments. These three opportunities for improving design for nature in dementia care will now be examined more closely, each followed by suggestions for implementation.

LOOKING OUT AND WATCHING

For a view to be successful it must appeal to its viewers, engage their attention and be satisfying on some level. Even though whether something is a good view is subjective and people will prefer different views, having a choice of good views that differ in content will satisfy a range of tastes. 'View content' concerns what is actually in the view – whether it be people, traffic, trees, gardens, the ocean or the car park. A view is also limited or enhanced by the location of a room within the building, and the location of the building within the landscape. Another aspect that affects one's view relates to the amount of time a person spends in any given room during the course of the day. And, lately (as you will read later in this chapter), through the use of assistive technology, people can have a 'window on the world' which offers the potential to view spaces normally beyond their reach.

Preferences over view content

Clearly, a view from a care environment has to satisfy a broad range of interests given the diversity of the residents cared for. So the view needs to be diverse enough to appeal to a group of people. One aspect of a view is that it grows less interesting over time, with the first view of something seeming to have a higher impact than subsequent viewings. Why this happens is unclear and is a matter that needs some research. However, is this actually true for people with dementia who might not remember having seen the view before?

Given these two aspects of a compelling view – that it needs to be diverse and that it needs to stay fresh and new – one approach is to offer views that are both diverse and changeable. A mixture of built and natural environment supplies a diversity of view content. In terms of providing visual interest from frequent movement, urban scenes change more quickly than green scenic nature scenes do. More peaceful scenes tend to be rural or scenes viewed from a distance. For people with visual impairment or diminished sight, movement and colour are also important aspects of view.

Research by the author (Chalfont 2006) in which people were interviewed while looking out of a window explored reasons why they found a view enjoyable. These included human activity in the street, as well as peaceful greenery. For example, one resident, Mary, was visually and physically impaired, but stood for a moment when returning from dinner to enjoy the view.

GC: What do you see?

Mary: Lovely trees and bushes… ah, it's beautiful… it really is beautiful, in't it… do you think it is?

GC: Yeah I do, it's a nice view isn't it?

Mary: Yeah it is… and it is a picture really, because, look at all these lovely beautiful trees, and look at these lot, people pass them and never look, don't they. They don't know what they're missing. They really don't. Lovely… I'd be standing up here, if I could stand… (laughs) and look.

GC: I don't blame you.

Mary: Well I mean it's nice isn't it. If you haven't got these things at home you might as well take advantage when you come here… mighten I?

Another resident, Sharon, could see the grassy bank from her upstairs bedroom window. Sharon's comments seemed to shed light on her personal feelings about her dementia.

Sharon: I like to see… Birds on the lawn, not a long time. They don't let themselves get poorly.

GC: Can you think of one kind you know?

Sharon: Ox…can't find… I know the names of all the birds. I like the lawn and I like the new people who make the lawn good.

GC: Do they come very often?

Sharon: Oh, yes. Well they follow a path. They do a lot of things. I bet most people like me will be better. I've forgotten where they were born. They go to a tree with a hole in it and they make a special… They stop there and look at their lives, proper skirts. They're looking for food, animals looking for food. They want to make it into a tree… Can't find the words …the word's gone and I know what it is.

Personal preference varied widely as to what view attracted and held a person's attention. A good strategy for planning views from a home would be to give people different view content (or content that changes throughout the day), being sure to include colour, diversity and movement.

Building floor plan and topography

The content and character of the view – and therefore the quality of the experience of looking out and watching – depends on the floor plan of the building and the positioning of the building in terms of its surroundings. The topography, or 'lay of the land', makes a difference because if the building is at the top of a hill, the view could be wide and distant. But if the building is at the bottom of a hill, the view may be foreshortened by a grassy bank or a brick wall. A room could be situated on the bottom floor or one higher up, and could also be looking towards the interior of the site or out towards the neighbourhood. Each of these locations would determine the potential views. A diverse view with active content would contain foreground, middle ground and distance, and a view to a busy area. Ideally, a room with a view would look out of the site and be in a part of the building unobstructed by topography.

Library
Knowledge Spa
Royal Cornwall Hospital
Treliske
Truro. TR1 3HD

Location of people during the day

Another aspect of looking out and watching relates to a person's usual position in the building and the amount of time he spends there throughout the day. As is often the case in a care environment, residents spent long parts of each day in one or two rooms (Chalfont 2006). This is especially true if people's mobility is limited, either through their own pre-existing physical disability or through institutionalised disability (for instance, lack of walking, or encouragement to sit down). People's experience of looking out and watching is affected positively or negatively, depending on the views available from the room and from the chairs when they are sitting in them.

Time–space mapping can be used to show where people spend time during the day and how much time is actually spent in which rooms. To do this, you should fit the floor plan of the building on to an A4 sheet of paper and photocopy it several times. Then mark on the sheets what time of day it is, and walk around the home marking the location of each resident at that particular time of day. Such 'time maps' should also include people being in the corridors and bathrooms and will thus give a clear picture of room usage at various times throughout the day. (For more on the use of mapping in outdoor environments see Hernandez (2007)). The views from the rooms that are used the most will have the greatest effect on people and should therefore be given most consideration. From a care perspective, rooms with the best views are the ones that should be used the most. If an architect has a choice about room placement in a care setting, a lounge rather than a dining room should have the better view, because people are likely to spend more time in this room.

Technology – webcam

The issues of looking out and watching also relate to the use of assistive technology to connect people to the larger community. (From 2003 to 2007 the INDEPENDENT Project researched domestic environments and the use of assistive technology for people with dementia. It was funded by the EPSRC (Engineering and Physical Sciences Research Council) and involved the Universities of Liverpool, Bath and Sheffield. Project partners included SheffCare, Northamptonshire Social Services, Huntley Healthcare and Dementia Voice.) In 2006 the Independent Project developed and trialled a 'Window on the World' device for people with dementia to enable connection to the wider world using webcam technology, a flat screen monitor, a two-button remote controller and two cameras (see Figure 4.1). During the trials the device was enjoyed by residents who looked out onto areas around the home they could not usually see. Using the remote control was quickly and easily mastered by people in the study, who found the technology fun and interesting.

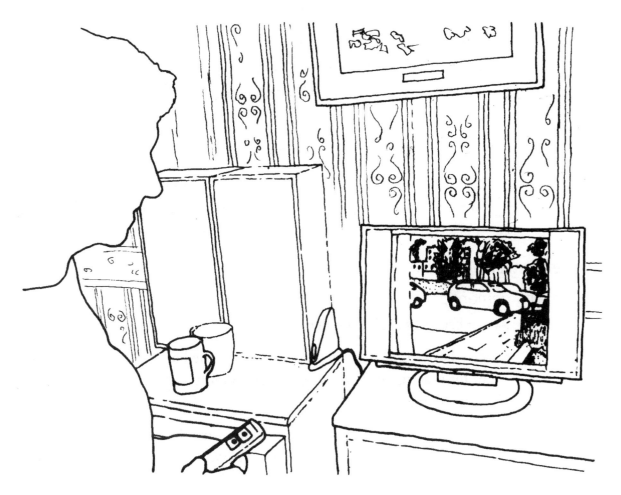

Figure 4.1 'Window on the World', UK

Using the 'Window on the World' was also useful for generating discussion and providing entertainment as people recognised and commented on who and what they saw on the screen.

A family care-giver involved in the INDEPENDENT Project had the following to say about it:

Melanie: It's a change off the television and it's something that should be more interesting to them… but this is actual happening here… Everybody likes to look out and to see things, otherwise it's boring, I mean it's all part of… making things interesting for them isn't it? You know, so to look even if they can only see vandals or whatever (chuckles), but it's there and they can… Might see people getting off the bus who they know… and it'll trigger off a conversation. You can say 'Oh yes, I know her, she used to live near me.' And that's what they need, isn't it, something to talk about, not just see, something to talk about, don't they?

GC: Another webcam is going to go in the car park.

Melanie: Oh, yes, so they'll be good to see us come in, won't they? And various people… you know if they see other people… It's all connected. They can see the bus when they come in if they're going on outings, and they can look about. They'll see people who go to the day centre… I think they would be able to register with this and say 'Oh yeah, if she's gone, and I've seen her go, then I would like to go today.' Yeah, I think this is a really good idea.

When the device was in use a resident said:

It's a lovely picture and all, you know, clear. Oh, it's not bad. Well it's different in't it? Showing you people, you know, what's what.

Implementation

Person with dementia

Remember that people with dementia:

- may have a preference in view content for the bustle of urban street life or for peaceful, rural scenery, or a person may simply need to see just something going on

- may spend large amounts of time on the same floor, in the same room, and even in the same chair, so their view will determine their levels of boredom or stimulation

- may be visually impaired, so a view must provide not just details, but aspects they may still be able to enjoy, such as colour, movement or the quality of light.

Social environment

- In homes where the care routine largely determines where people spend most of their time, consider whether the views from well-used rooms are diverse and contain active content.

- Consider changing the way a room is organised, the time of day it is used or which rooms are used for what activity, if this means improving people's view.

- Views can be a stimulating source of free entertainment and general discussion.

Physical environment

- Design for diverse and changing view content by positioning the building to include a range of outlooks – from the bustle of human activity to green scenic nature.

- Ensure that a diversity of views is available by increasing the number and location of windows and by enabling the use of different rooms in the building throughout the day.

- Avoid blocking views with the lay of the land or the building structure.

- Avoid views towards the interior of the site, if no action normally occurs there.

- Design for rooms where people spend the most time to have the best views.

- Install flat screen and webcam technology into care environments to afford residents a view to the wider world beyond their immediate space.

Message: Pay attention to a building's placement, the rooms where time is spent, the view content and any technology that can help people to look outside and watch.

INTEGRATING INDOORS AND OUTDOORS

At a building's edge lies an opportunity to integrate indoors and outdoors through design and use. This can be done by paying attention to natural light and the ways it enters the building, which is directly affected by the height and placement of windows. The location of furniture in relation to the windows will also determine both the amount of light received by people in the room and the views that will be possible. Aside from windows, further opportunities to integrate indoors and outdoors occur in entrances and balconies at the building edge. A relatively forgotten space in modern care environments is the covered walkway or cloister, which will be revisited as a way to enliven the edge.

Natural light

It is known that daylight is beneficial to human beings, but for people living in care environments, much of their time can be spent indoors where their only exposure to it is from daylight reaching into the building. The daily cycle of night and day, which includes both lightness and darkness, is also known as the 'diurnal cycle'. A common symptom of dementia is dislocation of diurnal rhythms, so people tend to be awake and active at night. The evidence is very strong that the absence of a clear day–night lighting cycle has a deleterious effect on health and this may be especially significant for people with dementia (Torrington and Tregenza 2007) (see text box 'Natural light and dementia').

In order for the body to regulate its diurnal cycle, as well as avoid the risk of Seasonal Affective Disorder, it is necessary to experience a 24-hour cycle of light and dark. Buildings should therefore have freely accessible internal areas with strong daylight that are used for normal daytime activities to ensure people actually benefit from light entering the building (Torrington and Tregenza 2007). Figure 4.2 shows a sunny seating area with tall windows to the south and west. The view includes the nearby houses, mature trees, a school and a playground.

Natural light and dementia

Research has shown that long-term care residents often live in conditions of inadequate lighting and frequently receive inadequate exposure to high-intensity light (Sloane *et al.* 2005). As well as low levels of light penetrating the building, the fact of people receiving little or no exposure to sunlight can be due to their limited mobility, a lack of access to outdoors, or inclement weather conditions (Campbell *et al.* 1988; Savides, Messin and Senger 1986). It is known that several physiological systems are triggered by daylight exposure, including secretions of melatonin and other hormones as well as a circadian pacemaker in the brain (Kryger, Roth and Carskadon 1989). As well as also supplying vitamin D, natural light is particularly important for people with dementia because they often suffer from dislocation of diurnal rhythms (Volicer *et al.* 2001). A disruption of these daily sequences of physiological change may result in depression and sleep disorder, and higher light levels have been shown to positively affect sleep, mood and behaviour in people with dementia (Forbes *et al.* 2004). Bright light treatment was also shown to treat sleep disorder and depression in people with dementia (Cheston and Bender 1999). Furthermore, Ancoli-Israel and Kripke discovered several light-related aspects of sleep fragmentation in people with and without dementia, noting that many nursing-home residents never experienced bright light at any point during 24-hour recordings (Ancoli-Israel and Kripke 1989).

Windows and furniture

The height of windows matters for a number of reasons. A seated person cannot see out of high windows, while low windows do not allow light to penetrate any distance into the room. A maximum windowsill height of 600mm (2 ft) or less will ensure that a person sitting in a chair or wheelchair is able to see out. Horizontal glazing bars (where the window panes join each other) should not intersect a person's view when sitting down, which should be unobstructed. This can be accomplished by using larger or vertical panes of glazing at the seated eye level. Windows also moderate privacy by determining what a stranger can see of the interior rooms from outside the building. Curtains and sheers, or lace curtains, are often used in residential settings to shield the person from

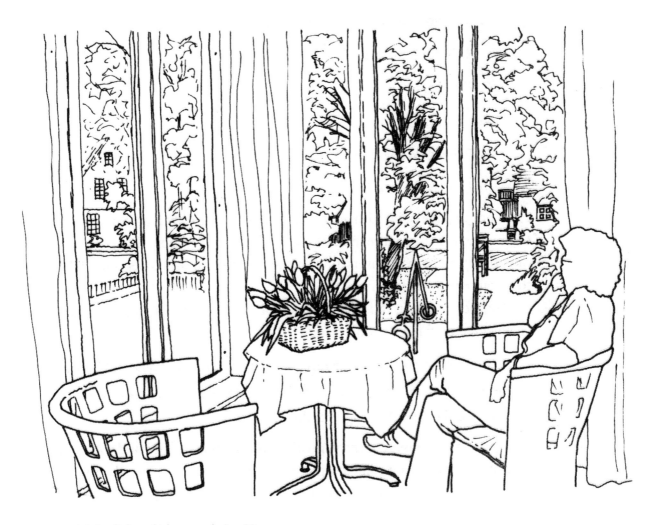

Figure 4.2 Daylight and playground view, Norway

outsiders looking in. They also facilitate the resident looking out without being observed, because they give a degree of privacy.

Another aspect of integrating indoors and outdoors is thoughtful placement of furniture to ensure that light actually reaches people sitting in the room. Furniture also determines to some degree the view that is possible. Furthermore, furniture placement has also been found to determine the potential for social interaction while viewing. The author's research into 'edge space' examined the use of nature for people with dementia during conversations. For the purpose of the study, edge space was defined primarily in terms of proximity to a window and availability of seating or standing room nearby – two elements that enabled a conversation to occur. (A good example of edge space appears in Figure 4.2.) Edge space provides people with dementia with a way to connect to others because nature provides the stimuli for conversations. In the following example, Dorothy was sitting with the author in the dining room looking out onto a grassy slope in the garden.

GC: Have you ever been up on top of that hill?

Dorothy: I don't think so. I think Tommy has but I haven't.

GC: Who has?

Dorothy: Tommy.

GC: Tommy? Who's Tommy?

Dorothy: Used to be with me.

From her vantage point in an edge space near the window Dorothy was able to see out and discuss a place. Both the view to the garden from the space and the opportunity to be in a conversation enabled her to mention somebody who used to be quite important to her.

Another resident, Nicole, was looking out from an upper floor and commented on what she observed.

> Cats is just on main road like this, like that one, and cats come and have a
> sleep on there, on that grass verge, or at night time, it's late, but they don't
> care and they're still going, cats do.

Seeing an empty grass verge prompted Nicole to discuss what cats do. A moment later she was observing something moving on the ground, blown by the wind, which prompted a series of questions.

> What's that? Blowing in grass. End of…what is it? It's blowing in grass at
> bottom now wi' a pink thing. Look, sun's on it. It's not a bird is it? Might
> be a toffee paper what's got a silver lining.

People with dementia taking part in the research were highly perceptive of nature outdoors and inquisitive of elements in their view. From the comments of Dorothy and Nicole, it is possible to see how views of nature played a role in stimulating their thoughts, and being in the company of an interested listener allowed them to communicate their thoughts. Furthermore, the physical availability of edge space made both the viewing and the social interaction possible. A more detailed account of the Edge Space Study, including conversations with five people with dementia, photographs, floor-plans of the locations where the conversations occurred, a literature review and a theoretical framework for the research, can be found in Chalfont (2007). It is also discussed in the text box 'The Edge Space Study'.

The important contribution of the Edge Space Study was not just in documenting these two interactions (person with nature, and person with person), but also demonstrating their potential, for it was the *combination* of these two interactions that enabled the person with dementia to engage in higher levels of communication. The whole was greater than the sum of the parts, and

---

The Edge Space Study

This study, conducted in 2006, found that edge spaces facilitated sensory stimulation and social interaction and assisted the ability of people with dementia to express themselves creatively, including:

- using nature symbolically, giving insight into the spiritual aspects of their experience of dementia

- using nature for ethical reasoning, introspection and personification.

Because edge spaces supported social interaction while affording natural stimuli, these informal dialogues enabled manifestations of selfhood. In summarising the Edge Space Study, we can say that people with dementia used nature as a tool to communicate, and as a result, contributed to their own well-being (Chalfont 2006). For a diagram of these interactions, see Appendix 1, the Prosentia Hypothesis (the term 'prosentia' was coined by the author to provide an antonym for the term 'dementia' and to draw attention to the potentially positive aspects of the disease from the person's perspective).

---

edge spaces enabled these two interactions to occur. They afforded sensory stimulation for the person with dementia, and they also supported conversation with another person.

The entrance and the balcony

The third aspect of integration between indoors and outdoors can be found in the wall itself, either at a ground level entrance or an upper level balcony. Entrances are transition zones. They can provide a sentry position, particularly if seating is provided, for watching people and traffic to find out what is happening in the outside world. Figure 4.3 has two good examples of entrance seating positions in a dementia-care home in Norway. The first position, labelled 'seating by the window', is the most popular indoor seating area. The outdoor area, labelled 'seating area by the front door', is a cool and shady location on warm days.

A balcony is a space at a level above the ground floor with fresh air, a view and seating (see Figure 4.4). A roll-down screen for shade from the afternoon sun also offers shelter from the breeze and privacy if desired. A balcony can be enhanced with plantings, especially if a staff member takes responsibility for hanging baskets and planters that need to be watered. A balcony (or 'veranda' in the UK) is described by one team leader in a focus group.

We've got a little veranda on the end there, haven't we, what's all fenced up and I used to do flowers. I used to do all the pots on there and they enjoyed that – looking at 'em. You can't see 'em now. I don't do it now because I'm not on that corridor, but I used to enjoy that and they used to like to come and help and we've potted sunflowers before, haven't we, things like that. You know, it's sweet peas trailing up the iron gate. It's all iron gated and we used to trail 'em all up and they used to come out and look at the colours and smells.

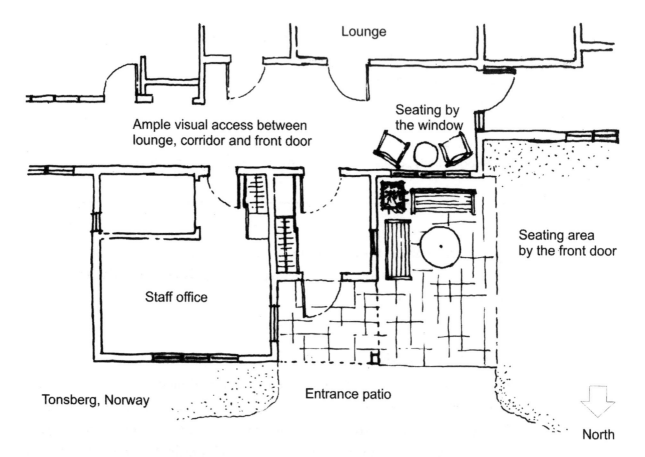

Figure 4.3 Entrance sentry position, Norway

Figure 4.4 shows a balcony on the south-west side of a building. Notice the rolled up blinds for shelter from the direct afternoon sun, the hanging plant and the view to the neighbourhood including nearby houses and the street.

Both an entrance and a balcony offer potentially more sensory stimulation from daylight, fresh air and views than do places further inside the home. Besides having these outdoor qualities they also extend the indoors by offering shelter and a vantage point. For instance, an entrance offers previews of the weather such as whether it is windy, and whether the ground is wet. Entrances also give older eyes time to adjust before going out, which is important as such eyes are more sensitive to glare (Grant and Wineman, 2007).

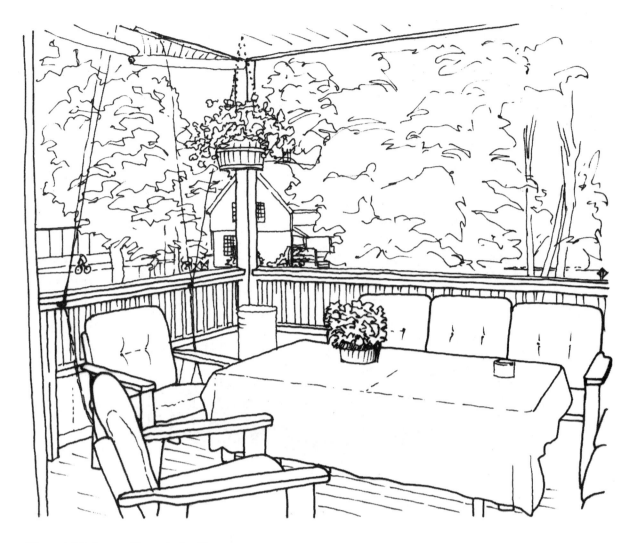

Figure 4.4 Balcony with sunshades, Norway

Depending on climate and culture, balconies and porches vary in size, how they are referred to, the extent of enclosure and the type of materials used, as well as their location within the building layout. A porch in the UK usually refers to a small room at the front door for hanging up coats and taking off muddy boots. A porch in the USA is a deck for outdoor living. Climatic variations on the balcony or porch affect their suitability for year round use, as well as the views that are possible. The main benefit of having a balcony or porch from the perspective of sensory stimulation and view is that it extends the comfort and security available inside the home, into a semi-outdoor space, where the stimulation from nature and the views of it can be more readily experienced.

Figures 4.5 and 4.6 show a Norwegian-style porch with an overhanging roof. This type of extended space can entice the inquisitive or curious person, and comfort the nervous or fearful person. This is especially possible when normal routine activities such as meals are carried out on it. A porch on either the rear or side of the home is more private and therefore appropriate for meals and snacks. The porch area can accommodate a barbeque grill as well as tables, chairs, hanging baskets, flower boxes and sun shades.

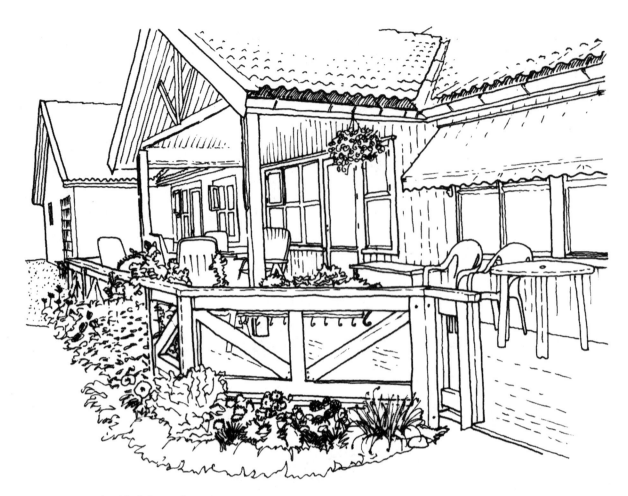

Figure 4.5 Porch with shelter and sun, Norway

Even an indoor space can be designed to look and feel like a porch, enabling porch-like behaviour such as sitting, looking out, greeting people and commenting on the action. Such a design has been incorporated into a 'sunroom' in an assisted living community (see Figure 4.7). This room makes good use of the space because it is positioned at an angle to the front entrance. Both pedestrian and vehicular traffic can be easily observed from this indoor sentry position. Windowsills are low and the room is only one storey high, which facilitates the use of skylights. The roof line and also the interior ceiling are sloped forward further, adding to the feel of a porch, even though the room is essentially an indoor space.

The use of rocking chairs is traditional on porches in many countries. They deserve wider use in dementia care as they have been shown to benefit psychosocial well-being and balance (Watson, Wells and Cox 1998).

The cloister and the ambulatory

The cloister and the ambulatory are not architectural terms one usually associates with modern care environments as they were features most commonly used in monastic buildings and churches. A cloister refers to a covered walk, with an open arcade or colonnade usually opening onto a courtyard but it can also mean

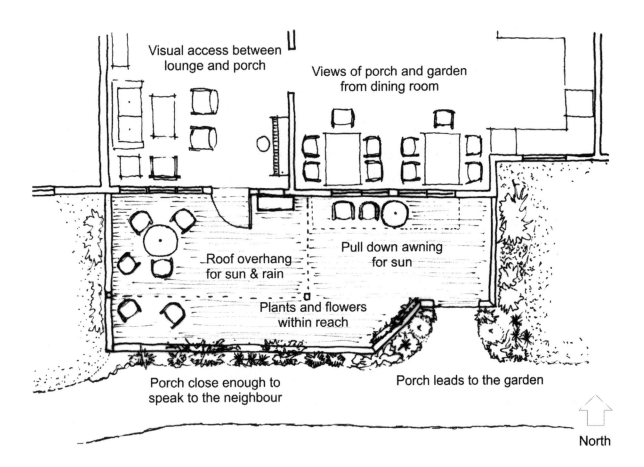

Visual access between lounge and porch

Views of porch and garden from dining room

Roof overhang for sun & rain

Pull down awning for sun

Plants and flowers within reach

Porch close enough to speak to the neighbour

Porch leads to the garden

North

Figure 4.6 Porch floor plan, Norway

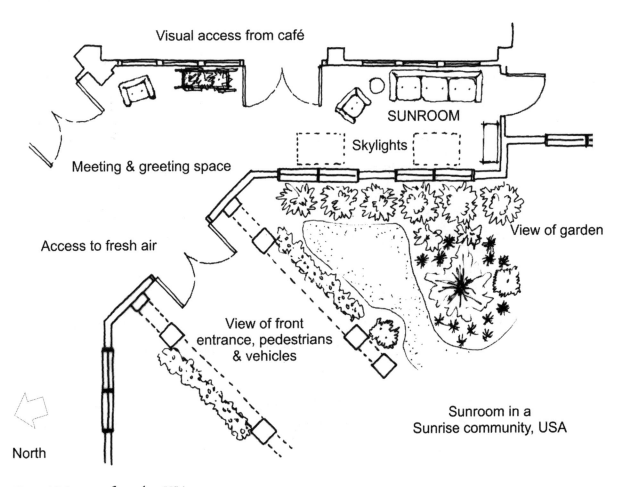

Visual access from café

SUNROOM

Skylights

Meeting & greeting space

View of garden

Access to fresh air

View of front entrance, pedestrians & vehicles

Sunroom in a Sunrise community, USA

North

Figure 4.7 Sunroom floor plan, USA

a courtyard bordered with such walks. The first documented example of a cloister garden designed for old and infirm people for fresh air, exercise and recuperation was on the St Gall plan of 820 AD, a Christian monastery in Switzerland.

The ambulatory is a covered walkway open usually on one side and attached to the wall on the other side. An ambulatory can also connect two buildings and be open on both sides. The benefit of the cloister and the ambulatory is that they offer an edge space where people can walk or sit at the outer wall of the building. Similar to the entrance, such spaces afford exposure to nature under the protection of the building, and, similar to the porch, they afford a space along the exterior wall. What the cloister offers is a walking or sitting space along the edge of a building and directly adjacent to a garden or lawn. A cloister also tends to connect in a circuit rather than have dead ends. What an ambulatory offers is a length of protected space where one can walk and exercise as well as take fresh air.

Although such spaces were documented in historic environments, few edge spaces reminiscent of the covered walkway exist in modern dementia-care environments today.

However, elements of this concept have been translated into the design of a wrap-around conservatory room (see Figures 4.8 and 4.9) in one dementia-care environment in the UK, offering a view to the garden in a sheltered space with two ways into the building.

Implementation

Person with dementia

Remember that people with dementia:

- may have limited mobility and will spend most of the day sitting, so they will need seating areas designed to optimally integrate the indoors and outdoors, and they will need the walls and windows designed to optimise their seated views

- may enjoy watching activity and being near the door, so they will need a choice of spaces to sit and stand near entrances

- need to receive sunlight on the skin every day in order to satisfy physiological needs for vitamin D and to moderate their sleep–wake cycles (circadian rhythms)

- need a choice in the levels of stimulation provided by the outdoor world and need opportunities to independently choose and access these various levels

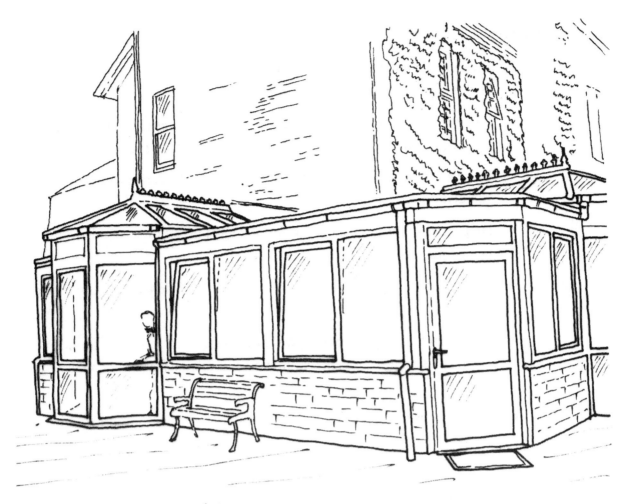

Figure 4.8 Conservatory wrap-around view, UK

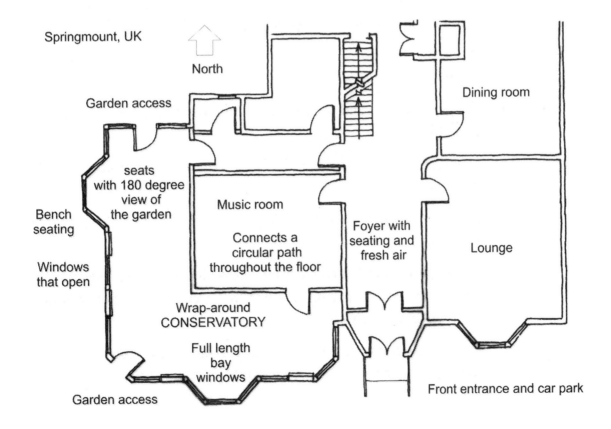

Figure 4.9 Conservatory wrap-around plan, UK

Social environment

- Facilitate communication for people by approaching them in edge spaces and engaging them in conversations about the view.

- Be aware of the potential natural sensations in the environment. What can be seen, heard or smelled from where the person spends time?

- Be aware of a person's sensory abilities when considering enjoyable stimulation.

- Help a person become aware of the elements of nature available to his or her senses.

- Plan for seating for two people to be available in close proximity to the windows.

- Place furniture by considering what the person can see while seated. Small adjustments can make a difference in the quality and content of the view.

- When choosing rooms to use during the day, consider good daylight levels.

Physical environment

- Locate living rooms in the building to take advantage of the natural light available at times of day when people will be using the rooms.

- Specify the furniture and its location in order that people can take advantage of the views.

- Design the height and placement of windows to take advantage of natural light.

- Avoid specifying windows with glazing bars at eye level when seated or standing.

- Design entrances to include seating for people to watch others coming and going.

- Design porches with a comfortable micro-climate that extends use through the year by paying attention to placement, extent of enclosure and type of materials used.

- Design a cloister or an ambulatory to provide semi-enclosed sitting and walking space adjacent to a garden or lawn area, for taking exercise and fresh air.

Message: Enliven the experience of nature for people with dementia by integrating indoors and outdoors with views, seating, entrances, porches, cloisters and covered walkways.

SUPPORTING WILDLIFE

A third way that can be used to increase people's experience of outdoor nature is to ensure the presence of wildlife in their living environment. This section explains how to support wildlife through the health, diversity and nearness of habitats and ecosystems, and the presence of wildlife in urban environments.

Habitat and ecosystems

A basic principle in supporting wildlife is that habitat is the essential requirement and thus to support birds, one needs to plant trees. Habitat provides the basics of food and shelter, and should provide niches and materials for nest building and foraging. Additionally, a habitat must also supply fresh water. There are three essential qualities of a habitat if it is to be enjoyed by a person in dementia care – it must be healthy, diverse and nearby:

- A healthy habitat supports a population by adequately providing these essential ingredients of food, shelter and water.

- Second, the more diverse the habitat, the higher number of species it can support.

- Finally, the nearer the habitat is to the buildings where people live, the greater the possibilities for people to actually see and hear the wildlife it supports.

During the author's research of edge spaces in residential care environments, some participants showed a freedom of expression in their ability to move between their present moment-to-moment experience and their long-term memories. From the analysis of data collected about the sensory elements in the environment during these conversations, it was suggested that it was the richness of sensory stimuli in the edge spaces that enabled such creativity to occur in their dialogue. Nicole is again looking out an upstairs window and remarks on the flowering tree, which then takes her thoughts to a bird that comes to visit it.

> Oooh, it's beaut… I think it's a shame to cut it down, and well they go for it and make two little, don't they. They make their friends like that and they fly on to one another. One mine, I got, uh. Oh what they call 'em now I've forgot? What did they call 'em? They're like black and white, and they're like, oh they can sing and they can skip and owt!

Urban environments

While rural locations more readily support wildlife through the availability of habitat such as farmland, woodland, hedgerows and ponds, establishing healthy, diverse and nearby habitat in urban environments can be a greater challenge. However, wildlife corridors, city gardens, green space and green roofs are some of the resources that are now contributing to the increase of wildlife habitat in urban environments, as well as addressing international environmental concerns such as global warming and air pollution. For care environments in urban areas it is even more crucial to contribute to habitat if at all possible, as the residents stand to benefit from having animals to watch.

Vertical structures such as trellises, walls and fences can make climbing frames for vines and can support a range of hanging baskets and bird houses. Window boxes, planters and pots can help to 'green up' an otherwise concrete barren space, and provide soil for a plant to put down roots and become established. Any foliage thereby created, if evergreen, affords the possibility that a bird may land on it or possibly nest in it. An expanse of pavement can be broken up by removing a small area of paving next to a wall, installing a trellis over it and planting an evergreen or a flowering vine in the hole. If an area of lawn is not being used it can be converted into habitat by sowing a 'pictorial meadow' with a flowering mix of native and non-native hardy annual seeds. This is an inexpensive and low-maintenance way to provide natural habitat, bio-diversity and scenic beauty from summer through to late autumn. This method is being used successfully on vacant land as an intermediary use between demolition and redevelopment on housing estates in the north of England, following years of trials at the University of Sheffield: see www.pictorialmeadows.co.uk.

To bring wildlife in and through the city, wildlife corridors can be created by mapping out the green spaces in the city, determining where the 'corridor' breaks down, and planting green spaces to link them up. Adopting an abandoned lot or even a small strip beside the road and planting it with species that provide nectar, berries or seeds can help connect a corridor and provide habitat. Wild areas that can be planted and left to go to seed in the autumn, rather than cut down and cleared away, will provide winter food for birds.

Creating habitat can also be done by building bird houses. This is an advantage to both birds and people if the bird house is visible from inside the home (see Figure 4.10). Although most birds prefer to nest in habitats they build themselves, some species of birds such as house martins and bluebirds will nest in bird houses if erected, even when these are close to buildings. Others, such as swallows, build their own nests from mud and are comfortable nesting near people. Bats are also wonderful creatures, with unfair reputations thanks to Hollywood! Bats have soft fur, expressive eyes and huge ears and can eat 600 mosquitoes in an hour. Bat boxes are cheap and easy to install and will encourage

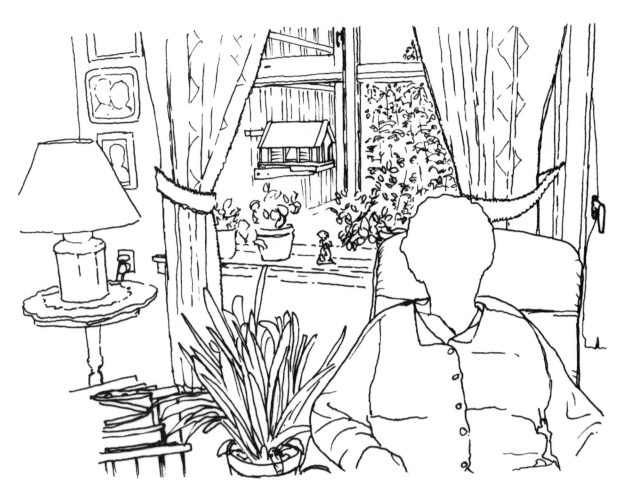

Figure 4.10 Bird house in window view, Norway

bats to live nearby. Watching them swoop fast and gracefully at dusk in a summer sky is a magical experience.

Although it is hard to imagine because they look so fragile, some butterflies are migratory and travel great distances. There are many websites that provide information on their habits and flight patterns, or a local butterfly enthusiast may be able to advise you. Habitat for butterflies consists of plants for nectar (umbelliferous varieties such as *verbena* and Queen Anne's Lace) and structural plants for laying eggs on such as ornamental grasses. Butterflies also have specific needs concerning water, mud puddles, warm stones and lack of wind. If proper habitat requirements for the butterfly life-cycle are beyond the ability of the site, butterfly bushes (*Buddleia*) grow anywhere, thrive on neglect and offer opportunities for viewing. Prune them back in late March or early April to encourage dense flowering and to keep them under control.

Habitats are also available along the water's edge, such as marsh, pond, beach or wetlands, and the habitat at the edge where the water meets the land is often rich in species diversity. But even man-made ponds with constructed walls can become home to more species over time if vegetation starts to take root around the edges, or if islands or platforms are installed for ducks. When a stream or river passes through a town or city it provides habitat for waterfowl, as well as the fish and insects that support them. Frogs are also easy to attract by simply building a small pond. In some countries, their melodious sounds on warm summer nights are an enchanting conversation piece.

A watershed is the large geographical area that drains into the same body of water. To determine which watershed you live in, imagine a raindrop and trace on a map the downhill journey it takes. So for instance, the San Francisco Bay watershed would encompass all the land which drains into the Bay. Management ordinances protect watersheds by 'retaining' rainwater close to where it falls, allowing it to slowly percolate back down through the soil to recharge the underground aquifers. Retention ponds on a building site hold runoff water and can be designed to provide habitat for waterfowl. These can also be a visual amenity for residents and visitors if the building is designed to take advantage of it. Two aspects to include in the design are physical and visual access. For instance, the plan should be designed to include gated access to a walkway around the perimeter with benches. A 'bluebird trail' (a series of bluebird houses installed along a path) can be built with help from local enthusiasts or the wildlife association. A daily escorted walk around the pond can help people develop their sense of place and feelings of stewardship for the landscape and its wildlife, as well as introduce fresh air and exercise into a daily regimen. If architects could plan for the pond to be visible from inside the home it could stimulate conversation. To prevent accidents, adequate supervision is required near water, as well as appropriate design precautions such as fencing and non-slip surfaces near the edge of the pond.

Greening cities is of global concern as trees and green spaces reduce the heat generated in built-up areas as well as improving air quality and supplying oxygen. Planting a tree, wherever possible, is therefore to be encouraged. Some tall narrow cultivars, including flowering varieties, grow well in remarkably little space. City gardens and green spaces that are nearby are valuable for fresh air, exercise and social opportunities, with bowling greens being especially enjoyable both for participating and watching. When greening of the ground is impossible due to complete lack of space, there is always the potential to green a roof. This can be designed into new buildings or an older building can be modified. Funding and grants are often available for sustainable and ecological modifications to buildings.

Some flat roofs, if not draining properly, will green up naturally and support moss and weeds, providing the beginnings of a soil layer that can support insects and thus attract birds. In one of the study homes for the Edge Space Study there was a naturally occurring green roof which was readily seen from an upper window because it was on a lower part of the building. Nicole was watching as a bird landed on the roof below.

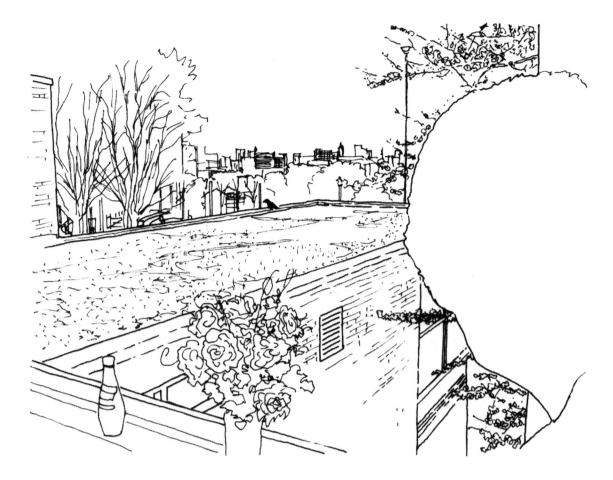

Figure 4.11 Flat roof attracts a crow, UK

Here look! Can you see it? It's my friend that. It's come for its finish grub haven't ya? Click, click, click. Come on! Click, click, click… Come on! Click, click, click. And look, he knows you've (indiscernible) down here (laughs). Should see him fly while… dear me (shouts) Come on! Come on little 'en! Here be! Here be! Come on… fly now…oh, there's…waiting for you on the wall yonder. It's a shame though the way they get nowt in't it? I give 'em some. Pretty! Come on ducky!

This is an example of how an unintentional habitat of a naturally occurring vegetated roof provided a person with wildlife interactions. Intentional green roofs can provide multiple benefits and could easily be designed into dementia-care settings. For more information visit www.livingroofs.org.

Implementation

Person with dementia

Remember that the person:

- may have been an avid birdwatcher and may still enjoy watching birds

- may have a rural or a farming background and may still identify with it

- may have encountered wildlife while camping, walking or backpacking

- will have little sense of attachment to the care environment and so will need ways to develop this if she is to feel at home to any degree

- may be able to enjoy a sense of purpose and must have opportunities to feel this.

Social environment

- Be aware and supportive of local habitat and bio-diversity initiatives, encouraging residents to sign a petition or write a letter in support of local wildlife sanctuaries.

- Involve residents in wildlife actions such as the national bird count by the RSPB.

- Involve care-givers in projects such as building a bird house.

- Enable residents to regularly put out water for the birds. It could be somebody's daily task to clean out the birdbath and refill it.

- Use, promote and take advantage of nearby natural resources, to help prevent them from disappearing. For instance, organise a trip to the nearby woodlands when the bluebells are in bloom, to the stream that meanders through the village to feed the ducks, or to the local fishing lake to count swans or spy the blue heron.

- Conduct a daily walk outside to foster stewardship, and provide opportunities for bird-watching and experiences to reflect upon later in the day.

- Involve residents in the creation and monitoring of a bluebird trail.

- Work towards an official designation of the garden area as a wildlife sanctuary.

Physical environment
Location or design of buildings and amenities

- Locate care environments near areas of natural resources, habitat and scenery such as woodlands, marsh, moors, pond, lake or sea.

- Design green roofs on new buildings or when modifying or renovating older ones.

- Position the buildings on the site with reference to habitat and natural resources, paying special attention to the views from rooms where people will spend most time – consider what they will see both on-site and in the borrowed landscape off-site.

- Align outdoor seating areas towards natural scenery.

- Encourage walking by designing short paths that can be used year-round.

- Provide a birdbath or a pond as a source of still water for wildlife.

- Design a water feature with flowing water such as a waterfall, or a small pond with an aerating fountain close to the home.

Improvement or maintenance of the natural environment

- During construction or renovation projects, if at all possible retain mature trees and habitat that already exist on site.

- Design a diverse landscape of trees, plants, flowers and evergreen vines, using deciduous, flowering, perennial and annual varieties which contribute to habitat (don't stay limited to the usual institutional landscape plants).

- To increase habitat on existing sites, plant a mixture of evergreen and deciduous trees and bushes, ground cover, vines and herbaceous perennials.

- Plant species for birds that offer fruit, nuts and seeds, such as berries, soft fruits, nut bushes and ornamental grasses.

- Plant perennial flowers and herbs. Allow them to go to seed and remain over the winter to provide food, cover and nesting materials for birds.

- Plant new, and retain existing, evergreens and conifers for year-round habitat.

- Encourage wildlife by keeping brush piles, wood piles and thickets on site and undisturbed, thus providing habitat in which to hide, nest, forage and feed.

- Encourage year-round nesting places for birds by growing evergreen vines on walls and trellises. (Do not allow vines such as ivy to grow up into trees.)

Message: Cultivate wildlife on the ecosystem level with habitats and green spaces so care home residents' daily lives contains stimulation, interaction, fresh air, exercise and a sense of place.

Chapter 5

Activities Outdoors

INTRODUCTION

The second part of this book began by looking at the natural world outside and at ways to enhance a person's experience of outdoor nature through design of the built and social environments specific to dementia care. This chapter turns the focus onto people themselves, their activities outdoors and the design require-ments of the care environment to facilitate these. The subject of outdoor activities can be broken down into a spatial progression of involvements. In other words, various activities fit into a continuum of spaces – from a person's activity close to the door, to a person taking a trip out of town. Within this sequence, the wide range of abilities and resources involved is systematically discussed.

Simply going outside, taking a walk or sitting in the garden stimulates the senses, supports well-being and encourages interaction (Rappe and Topo 2007). We might consider such activities to be less physically challenging and more passive than gardening, domestic activities or taking a trip. However, for a person with dementia, what constitutes a challenge is more than the physical. What challenges someone is highly individual and depends on many factors including his personality, fitness and mobility, tolerance for stimulation, fears and anxieties, the time of day, the social support available and the specific effects of dementia on that person. How 'accessible' the care environment is will depend on its ability to respond to a person with very complex needs. This chapter will look in particular at six outdoor activities and, using what people with dementia have said and done, will provide insights into these needs. The activities are: going outside, taking a walk, sitting in the garden, gardening, domestic activities and taking a trip.

GOING OUTSIDE

This seemingly simple act can be a great challenge in dementia care. There are the basics of physical accessibility to consider, such as handrails, door widths, ramps, turning radii and stopping-off places along paths. For design guidance on such issues consult the following publications: Centre for Accessible Environments (1998), Department of Health (2002) and Robson, Nicholson and Barker (1997). There is also design guidance for outdoor spaces for people with dementia given in Brawley (2006), Calkins (2005), Cohen and Day (1993), Judd, Marshall and Phippen (1998), and Tyson and Zeisel (1999). However, there is still a pressing need for further evidence-based research showing which design elements particularly facilitate use of outdoor areas and the benefits people with dementia can receive.

Post-occupancy evaluations can determine if outdoor places are actually used by the people they are intended for. For instance, in their 'Garden-use Model', Grant and Wineman (2007) identify five main categories of elements to enable effective use of outdoor areas: organisational policy, staff attitudes, visual access, physical access and garden design. Some of the specific factors that seemed to encourage outdoor use included: a variety of seating near the entry; legible circulation conducive to wayfinding; manageable doors; no change in elevation at entries; covered areas outside entries; unlocked doors and doors propped open; and the programming of outdoor activities. One interesting finding was that in two of the facilities, shady semi-private niches with seating tucked away from the building were a favourite destination, second only to seating adjacent to the building on a patio or terrace.

Climate and weather also affect outdoor use by frail older people who tend to feel the cold more easily, and who cannot move quickly if they are uncomfortable. Attention to temperature is not just about clothing but everything a person touches outside. For instance, handrails and seating must not conduct heat or cold. Metal handrails and furniture are tricky to get just right. A cool, metal handrail in the shade on a hot day can be pleasant, but once the sun moves around the metal can become red hot. Likewise, a warm metal arm of a bench in a sunny spot on a cool autumn day is also pleasant. But as soon as the sun goes behind the cloud the metal goes cold. But for an older person with dementia, these climatic considerations are even more complex. For some people their sensory perceptions are intensified, while other people may not be able to make sense out of the stimuli, and so might not feel the heat or cold. Although we don't want to wrap people up in cotton wool by creating environments that are deprived of intense sensory stimulation, the design of outdoor fixtures and fittings must be specific to the needs, frailties and cultural expectations of older people, to the climate and weather, as well as to their individual sensory perceptions.

But physical accessibility and thermal comfort aside, simply stepping outside for a person with dementia may seem an insurmountable hurdle or of no interest at all. This hesitancy can be overcome if that person's specific needs are addressed and if any resistance is seen as logical, and interpreted within the context of the physical environment and the care practice. This section will present some sensory, emotional and psychological issues related to going outside, drawn from the author's observational research.

Incentive and purpose

In order to encourage someone to go outdoors, it is helpful to develop incentives or purposes with which a person can easily identify. Simple pleasures reside in long-term memory – a warm sunny day, an ice-cream cone, a barbeque, smelling the roses, petting the cat, sitting in the sun, drinking a glass of wine and reading a good book… These words, we hope, conjure up images of pleasurable experiences for those hearing them. The particular images and words that resonate for someone are likely to emerge from him or her during conversations with family members or during interactions with other residents.

It is also quite possible for a person with dementia to develop new memories, especially if an experience has emotional content, such as laughter, excitement or romance, and if it also involves pleasurable sensation. One activity that has met with some success is to have the local ice-cream vendor bring the van into the parking lot (see Figure 5.1). Residents enjoy the opportunity to come

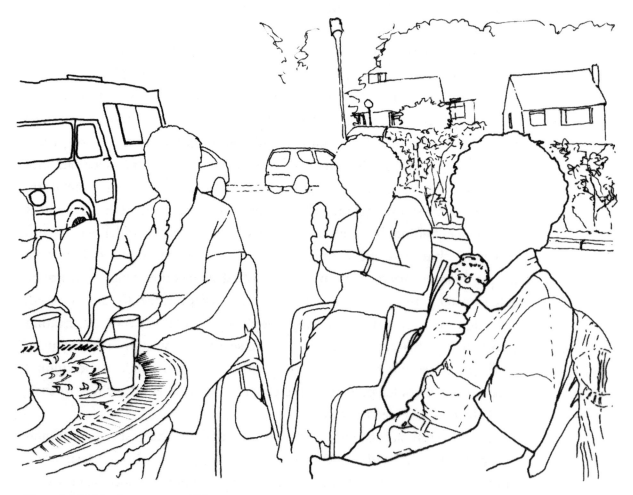

Figure 5.1 Visiting ice-cream van, UK

outside and to be a customer. This arrangement is mutually beneficial to the home and the vendor, costs the home nothing, and stimulates a great deal of social interaction, as well as providing sunshine and fresh air. Thus having places to sit outside makes the effort of creating them worthwhile.

Reasons for not going outside

Family care-givers often find it difficult when their loved one no longer wants to do things they once loved doing. For instance, it is common for residents to turn down an invitation to go outdoors, even if they used to love to go outdoors. 'No love, I'm alright. Not bothered.'

This is very common. Possible strategies for dealing with this include:

- asking her again later or when somebody else is also going

- asking her when a specific activity is going to occur

- asking her when she is already up and moving about

- asking for her help with a specific task

- when a family care-giver is able to join in, having the care-giver invite her

- consulting www.dementiapositive.co.uk for further resources for communication.

However, it is also not uncommon for a person with dementia to turn down a direct request to do something, especially if it involves leaving the room he or she is in. It is also not unusual for him or her to have a change of heart if the question is rephrased. For instance, he or she may be more willing to go if someone offers a hand and says, 'Let's go have a look at the garden, Bob', or, 'Are you coming with me, Anne?'

Other aspects are relevant to the physical environment. For instance, the person with dementia may be afraid to leave the room in case he misses a visitor. 'Me dad'll be coming for me.' There may also be psychological implications, depending on the 'time frame' in which the person feels he or she is living (Chalfont 2005a). For instance, if a person believes her father will be coming to pick her up, then her 'time-frame identity' is that of a younger person. The implications of being missing (for instance by being outside in the garden) if a parent comes to collect her might in her mind be severe, and certainly would not be worth the risk. It is therefore logical to her to turn down offers to go outside under these circumstances. In that particular case it would also be a design issue because it will help residents if they can see visitors arriving even if they are outside. In fact, if visitors entered the home from the outside area this could be an incentive for residents to use these areas.

There is another design issue in the fact that many outdoor areas are not visible from the indoor lounges. This can mean that when people are asked if they want to go outside, if they cannot see it, they may not know where 'outside' actually is, and may simply turn down a request to visit some unknown place. The evidence for this lies in the comments some people with dementia have made about different parts of the home – parts that do not actually exist. For instance, people with dementia may think they are in a building they remember from some time previous, perhaps a day centre they routinely visited before moving into care. They therefore have a mental map of that building. If that building had an outside area that was a long distance to walk, was always cold, had uncomfortable seats, or there was always a person there who they particularly disliked then these would all be reasons to resist going. So when Mrs T turns down an invitation to go outside, she may be turning down an invitation to go to an 'outside' she remembers negatively, not the outside that exists here and now. In design terms this suggests that all outside areas for people with dementia should be visible from inside the home, so it is clear which 'outside' is being discussed. Visual access is necessary if people are to clearly see where an entrance will lead to.

People with dementia will always be affected by such emotional and psychological factors that the disease creates, but there are also environmental aspects that will help to reinforce these perceptions. We cannot talk a person out of such beliefs, but we can design so that the social and built environments are not reinforcing them. For instance, if a person believes she is of school age, the care environment may be contributing to this false belief by the fact of it being a communal setting. This may be reinforced by the fact that people are called by their first names, meals are served communally, the day is run on a schedule, there is a bulletin board giving the day, date and year and what is on the menu, and a group of people are living together who are not related. This can appear very much like school or camp. Also, the room the person spends most of the day in can often resemble a waiting room. So it is little wonder that a resident might think a parent is coming to collect her from such an environment.

Fitness and mobility

The importance of exercise for people of all ages is evidence-based and much publicised nowadays. There is even evidence of an association between regular exercise and lowered risk for dementia later in life (see text box 'Exercise and dementia'). However, some care environments would seem to be contributing to physical disability by their emphasis on safety and avoiding risk. For instance, by eliminating a challenge such as stairs, a person's legs can 'forget' how to walk on stairs. In some care environments outside areas will be closed off if there is any danger that a person may trip and fall. So as people no longer walk on any surface other than level carpet, they lose the ability to do so. Ramps are even uncommon so that bit of exertion is also lost.

Exercise and dementia

Exercise is associated with reduced risk for incident dementia among persons 65 years of age and older (Larson *et al.* 2006). In a study of 1740 persons over 65 without cognitive impairment, the incidence rate of dementia was 13.0 per 1000 person-years for participants who exercised three or more times per week compared with 19.7 per 1000 person-years for those who exercised fewer than three times per week. The interaction between exercise and performance-based physical function was therefore statistically significant. When potential confounders were adjusted for, this corresponded to a 32 per cent reduction in risk for dementia.

Conclusion: These results suggest that regular exercise is associated with a delay in onset of dementia and Alzheimer's disease, further supporting the value of exercise for elderly persons.

After hours of sitting with little or no exercise, people's legs can swell and the only shoes they can then wear are slippers, often slit open. These give no support and are not appropriate for walking outside on concrete, asphalt or paving, and this may also be keeping people inside. A regime of no exercise, limited mobility, and keeping people seated in the belief that it prevents people falling, results in a downward cycle of diminished agility, strength and balance. Logically, the less people move about, the less they are *able* to move about, and the greater the possibility that they will fall from sheer lack of physical conditioning and muscle tone (see text box 'Exercise and MMSE').

Some of the specific benefits of regular exercise for people with Alzheimer's disease according to the Australian Government (www.betterhealth.vic.gov.au) include:

- reduced likelihood of constipation, reduced risk of falls because of improved strength and balance, reduced rate of disease-associated mental decline

- maintenance of motor skills

- improved mood, memory and behaviour

- better sleep and better communication and social skills.

'Use it or lose it' is a simple truth. Keeping people from moving to prevent them from falling may be having the opposite effect. This phenomenon is more damaging for people with dementia who already find it difficult to go outside, for reasons discussed above. To further remove the incentive by constantly being told to sit down will decrease the likelihood that they will go outside independently. (The only other places in which adults are instructed when and where to sit down are in a church or a doctor's office.) So, both the care and the physical environments can be helping to disable people with dementia, and by so doing, are reducing their contact with the natural world and contributing to an unhealthy life-style.

Exercise and MMSE

An interesting study in Brazil showed that MMSE (Mini-Mental State Examination) scores actually declined slightly from lack of exercise while it increased ever so slightly in the exercise group. Forty nursing-home residents took part in a controlled trial, at the end of which, the exercise subjects showed significant performance improvement in quantitative and qualitative obstacle-course scores, lower-limb function test, gait velocity test, knee extensor strength, and the GDS (Geriatric Depression Scale: a basic screening measure for depression in older adults), while the non-exercise subjects showed significant decrease in qualitative obstacle-course score, lower-limb function, gait velocity, MMSE, and the GDS (Bastone and Filho 2004).

Conclusion: This study strengthens the evidence that exercise is beneficial by indicating that there is a correlation between not only exercise and physical functioning (which one would expect) but also between exercise and improvements in cognitive performance and emotional well-being.

There are two dementia-related aspects of physical activity and exercise in care environments that have negative implications for going outdoors. One is the belief on the part of many people with dementia living in residential care that they are 'only visiting'. It is possible to understand people turning down an invitation to go outside and being content to just sit, if they think that they are going home soon and will resume an active lifestyle when they do. 'Why go outside now if I am going home soon anyway, and I can go outside with my husband in our own garden? Also, if I go outside the day-centre minibus might leave without me' (if they believe they are attending a day centre rather than living here).

Related to this belief is another one commonly held by participants in the Edge Space Study, that they were still living an active life. When asked, 'How do you spend your day?' a gentleman with severe mobility impairments who rarely leaves the building replied, 'Go out walking a lot.' 'Do you?' 'Yeah, I do.' Dorothy, who in reality also rarely went outside, gave this response:

GC: When do you go out into the garden?

Dorothy: I go out many a time of day. Walk through garden and have a look at things.

GC: Do you go out into the garden on your own?

Dorothy: Sometimes I walk round it if it's a nice day.

GC: Did you go out with somebody else?

Dorothy: Nobody to go out wi' when everybody's gone to work. So I have a walk round on me own.

The two beliefs cited above seemed to contribute to the general lack of physical activity in these people with dementia, and also to their reluctance to go outside. As this study lasted three years, long-term decline in physical conditioning was noticed among more than half of the participants, although not confirmed empirically.

Routine use

Making an outdoor activity part of a routine can help it seem less of a challenge. If a person does an activity regularly or has done it before, it can become familiar and the place where it occurs can seem less alien. There can be drawbacks to routines (that they stifle spontaneity and creativity for instance) but there can also be advantages in terms of outdoor usage, because once a routine is established a person generally expects it and may accept it. (This is not, however, true of routines some people may find unpleasant such as bathing, which they may consistently resist even though they have come to expect it.) The challenge is not only to ensure that going outdoors is a pleasure, but to make it expected – to establish a routine, pick a time of day and develop a pattern of going to a nearby space or taking a certain route, which people can then come to expect. It can help to make a video of these people using the outdoor areas enjoyably, in particular capturing their voices expressing joy or pleasure in the sights and sounds of the environment. This video can be played as a warm-up to going outside as a reminder of the benefits of doing so.

A study by Hernandez (2007) found that routines or 'rituals' played a role in how often the outdoor environment of a dementia special care unit was used. Rappe and Topo (2007), while investigating outdoor access in two dementia-specific day centres in Finland, found that visiting outdoors was a daily routine and the schedule for each day was organised to allow this. Participants took a walk either upon arriving at the centre or just before going home. This facilitated taking shoes and outdoor clothing on and off, thereby motivating those participants with low initiative to join in the walk. In one of the day centres, each person was taken for a walk individually in order for the staff person to have time to concentrate on that particular individual's well-being. In six residential units in the same study they found that being outdoors was a continuity of lifelong habits.

Implementation

Person with dementia

Be aware that people with dementia:

- may remember simple pleasures in terms of a nearby outside place that brought them enjoyment

- may be disinclined to go outside for sensory, emotional and psychological reasons concerning their dementia, fitness, mobility and memories

- may be in a downward spiral of limited mobility reinforced by lack of exercise, poor condition, diminished strength, agility and balance, resulting in a disincentive to go outdoors and reinforced by being told to sit down

- may believe they are visiting the facility rather than living there, and may turn down invitations to go outside, thinking that they are going home soon anyway

- may believe they maintain an active lifestyle when they are at home and therefore may turn down suggestions to go out for a walk or to exercise at the care home.

Social environment

- Ensure the person will be physically comfortable and warm when going outside.

- Organise for a person to enjoy simple pleasures such as ice-cream and sunshine.

- Invite the local ice-cream vendor to park outside at a certain time each week.

- If a person's history indicates that he enjoys going outdoors but response to an invitation to do so is negative, be inventive and flexible in how you phrase the invitation.

- Examine how often a person is encouraged to stay seated and consider if that may be having a negative impact on the person's physical mobility.

- Encourage movement, stretching, dancing, Tai Chi and going for walks to develop strength, flexibility and stamina.

- Pick a time of day and a certain route and destination and develop a daily routine.

- In a day centre, include a routine walk into the beginning or the end of the day.

- Video residents enjoying the outdoor areas as a reminder of an experience they have enjoyed.

- For tips on healthy living and activities visit www.healthyliving.gov.uk.

Physical environment

- Determine *when* outdoor areas can be used during the day and locate seating, furnishings and shelter to take advantage of the outdoor conditions at that time.

- Determine *what* outdoor areas can be used for (reading, sunning, people-watching, playing music, painting, sleeping, etc.) and furnish and use them accordingly.

- Ensure through use and placement of indoor furniture that outdoor areas are seen.

- Use distinctive plants, arbors, seating or sculpture along paths and at destinations.

- Use informal out-of-the-way seating for people to get away and find on their own.

Physical environment (specific to design professionals and commissioners)

- When positioning the building footprint, consider the outdoor areas the building mass will create as a result. Consider *where* areas are located and what sun, shade, shelter and micro-climate they offer at times when they are likely to be used during the day, and how big the window of possibility is for year-round use.

- Design interior spaces (rooms and corridors) with visual access to outdoor areas and at a minimal walking distance to the doors opening onto outdoor areas.

- Design paths and destinations with attractive and comfortable features.

- Meet basic physical access needs through Part M of the building regulations (ODPM 1999) and the needs of people with dementia through dementia-specific design guidance.

- For outdoor use during cooler weather, design seating areas that use the building mass, surrounding walls, trellises or raised beds to capture, reflect and retain heat.

- Specify furnishings and handrails that do not conduct heat or cold. (Tubular metal handrails need rubber coating, or wooden or plastic horizontal elements.)

- Build in physical challenges such as steps beside a ramp to offer people a choice, rather than inflict easiness upon the more able-bodied people.

- Create some outdoor areas that require effort to reach, so people are not deprived of opportunities to exert themselves, but maintain their physical ability to do so.

Message: Ensure that people with dementia enjoy the pleasures of going outside by fully understanding and addressing the issues that logically prevent them from doing so.

TAKING A WALK

To step outside and take a walk is a basic human right we all hope to retain throughout our lives. However, for people with dementia, the need to walk may go unmet if the right to walk is taken away from them. We have a duty of care towards these people and we also want to improve their quality of life. But, as discussed earlier, sometimes there are conflicting issues, such as safety versus freedom, and risk versus autonomy. There are also issues affecting wayfinding, such as the physical environment or the condition of paths and surfaces, and considerations about what people with dementia need and expect from neighbourhoods and destinations, and how these may have changed over their lifetime. There are also practical reasons for not taking a walk that are tied to the local geography as well as care practice. For instance, the need to go to the shop or the post office may diminish drastically once a person goes to live in care. Such changes can create bewilderment and anxiety and each of these aspects needs to be interpreted within the current reality of the person with dementia, who will need support in this both from care-givers and the physical environment (see text box 'Walking and exercise').

James McKillop, a person living with dementia, tells us that:

> when I was laid low with a back complaint, I found my short-term memory
> and my powers of reasoning and deduction fell away quite drastically. My

feet need to keep me in community circulation so that my mind is continuously stimulated. (McKillop 2006, p.104)

Walking and exercise

There are numerous positive reasons for walking, whether physical, social or cultural, including going somewhere, meeting people, talking things over with someone, getting some exercise, clearing the mind, doing an errand, walking the dog, going on a 'walkabout' or just getting out of the house. Voluntary exercise can improve physical health, increase learning and mental performance and increase brain plasticity (Cotman and Berchtold 2002). Exercise 'may have a beneficial effect on the mental processes...so physical activity should benefit mental processes as well as muscle strength, joint flexibility and balance' (Oddy 2006, p.74). So 'every person with dementia should be given a personal physical exercise programme' (Oddy 2006, p.78).

There is also interest in what has been called 'spirited walking', which extends the importance of spirituality in dementia care beyond the simple religious components such as denomination, priest or chaplain. Where 'spirituality is understood as the essence of a person, other paths will open up, inviting the carer to walk beside the person who has dementia, discovering together this person's unique spirit' (Hudson 2006).

Walking is something we can do with a friend or a dog. Not everyone likes dogs but for those who do, dogs are particularly good walkers as they facilitate regular routine outings into the local area and physical activity, while giving the person companionship, an added sense of security and increased independence (McColgan 2006). During recent interviews exploring the relationships between people and their dogs, participants said that 'by going on walks with their dogs they met other people, and that the dogs often acted as a catalyst for conversation' (McColgan 2006, p.108).

There can be further limitations to walking for a person with physical frailty or disabilities. Nonetheless, for one woman who was unable to walk very far and who used a walking frame for even short distances, the idea of taking a walk still resonated with a sense of freedom. She told her daughter she was going to go for a long walk, even though when her daughter invited her to go outside she felt it was too cold.

One significant change currently underway in dementia care stems from the ongoing recognition of the broader role walking plays in our lives. As a result, design is being approached with renewed enthusiasm and inspiration, focusing on how opportunities for movement can be created (Bennett 2006) (see also text

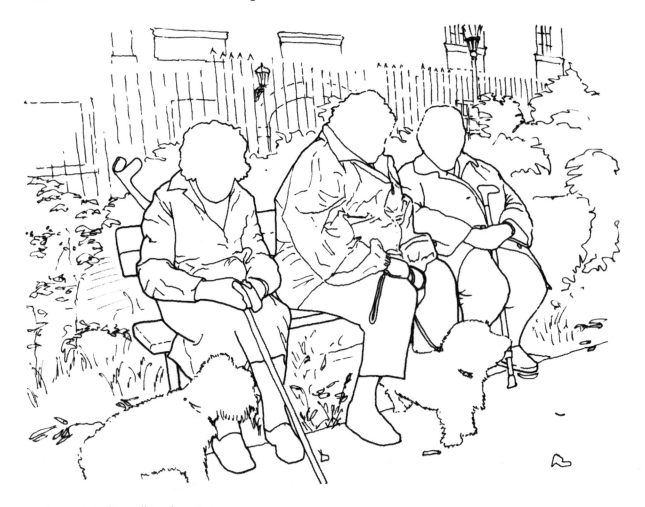

Figure 5.2 Ladies walking dogs, Prague

box 'Walking and dementia'). This broader, more positive understanding will affect how both the physical and social aspects of care environments are conceived and designed. The next section raises some research-based insights in this area and offers some guidance on it.

Safety and freedom, risk and autonomy

There are numerous reasons why a person with dementia living at home may be assessed for possible residential care (for example, forgetting to eat, bathe, change clothes or take medication), but if he or she walks out at night and forgets the way home, that often swiftly expedites a move into care (McShane, Hope and Wilkinson 1994; Wilson 2006). Few communities today are designed, either physically or socially, to enable safe outdoor movement for vulnerable people. There are many normal healthy reasons for walking, but when a person with dementia walks, it is often pathologised and termed 'wandering' (Marshall and Allan 2006) – which implies 'aimless and without purpose'. There can also be other reasons for walking such as boredom, discomfort, feeling lost and through time confusion (Alzheimer's Society

Walking and dementia

Various studies have found that walking and strength training for people with Alzheimer's and related dementia have measured improvements in chair-rise time, standing time, distance walked and walking speed, night-time sleep, agitation, mental function, capacity to communicate, continence and nutritional status. People in walking groups could walk significantly longer compared with their baseline performance than those in the control group who were not in a walking programme (Tappen *et al.* 2000). However, another study found that a walking programme produced no effect on ambulation (Cott *et al.* 2002). Preliminary findings in other studies suggest that walking and light exercise appear to reduce wandering, aggression and agitation (Holmberg 1997; Namazi, Gwinnup and Zadorozny 1994). In another study a psychomotor activation programme had significant beneficial effect on cognition but tended to increase rebellious and negative behaviour (Hopman-Rock *et al.* 1999).

2000), or underlying medical reasons such as depression or sleep disorder (Manning 2006). Marshall and Allan's book *Walking not Wandering* (2006) has raised awareness about why people walk and the possible meanings of walking for a person with dementia. This book encourages all those involved in the care of people with dementia to adopt constructive and helpful responses towards people who feel the need to walk, so as to improve their quality of life. Great benefit can be gained from reading this authoritative and useful rethink of 'wandering', from which this section benefited. The UK Wandering Network (UKWN) is also a good source for events, resources, tools and publications (www.wandering network.co.uk). See also the text box 'Wandering'.

The perspective of wandering as being 'challenging behaviour' currently informs the physical design and social management of care environments, with common responses to it being the control and restraint of physical movement, both indoors and out. In this context there is a role for careful and systematic assessment of behaviour (Allan 1994) as a way towards making more person-centred interventions and approaches that enable rather than undermine autonomy. Rather than making assumptions about the meaning and the motivation behind the behaviour, Stokes (2006), for example, advised that 'wandering' is a challenge not so much because of the behaviour itself, but in what it communicates about the unmet needs of the person.

The causes of wandering can be viewed from various perspectives (such as the physical, psycho-social and biomedical and that of human–environment interaction (Lai and Arthur 2003)), and a needs-driven approach to design for walking can be helpful in considering the experience of the person impacted by

---

Wandering

A systematic review of non-pharmacological interventions to prevent wandering found some evidence that exercise programs and multi-sensory environments in the form of light and sound relaxation sessions can reduce wandering and restlessness, but the studies supporting these techniques were of poor quality. They concluded that safe walking should be promoted rather than discouraged in people with dementia (Robinson *et al.* 2006). Tools are available such as the 'wandering' assessment process developed by the Dementia Services Development Centre at the University of Stirling (Allan 1994) and also the Bradford Dementia Group's 'Well-/ill-being' (WIB) profile (Bruce 2000) to 'enter into a person's world, make their actions more explicable and to help find out what might be driving a person' (Wey 2006).

---

factors across these various perspectives. For instance, a person's physical and sensory discomfort may result from noise, glare, air quality, heat and lack of exercise, all of which can be addressed through design. Their psychosocial distress might result from a lack of privacy or defensible space, or having no choice of rooms where one can exert some control over one's human contact. Equally, spatial design may include too much separation, resulting in someone's social exclusion and disconnection from the larger community. Wandering behaviour has often been attributed to boredom (Allan 1994), which may be a result of low levels of mental stimulation from having nothing to watch or do. Design solutions here could include having a view of the playground of a primary school, providing a shed or workbench for meaningful occupation, or the provision of useful furniture to enable creative activities – chairs around a table instead of chairs around a room. Wandering may also indicate that the person with dementia is searching for something. This could be considered a design issue too as such spiritual distress no doubt in part results from living in places devoid of meaningful attachment.

Personal and social approaches to wandering

First, and perhaps most importantly, it has been said that, 'The key to best management of wandering behaviour is to allow the person to walk freely and to destinations of interest without subjecting them to unnecessary risk or causing unnecessary distress' (Lyons and Thomson 2006, p.53). Physical barriers or technologies 'may help to minimise risk or distress, but only in conjunction with good design of the living environment, stimulation and activity appropriate to the individual and appropriately trained caregivers' (Lyons and Thomson 2006, p.53). 'Poor design can also be the cause of significant psychological abuse for a person who is searching for the past or who feels they have a job to perform' (Ferguson 2006, p.56). To enable a person to walk with a sense of freedom in an environment of lowered risk requires an overall programme of well-being, that integrates personal and social as well as physical approaches. Examples of social approaches include:

- stitching a name and a phone number into the pocket of a person's coat

- enabling the person to join a walking club, or

- training a companion dog to go with the person who knows the way home.

The personal approach is to go walking with the person when she needs to go.

Physical approaches

Physical approaches to the issues of wandering involve design that affords freedom of movement with minimal risk. For instance, it is important to highlight areas where a person is allowed to go and downplay areas that are not directly relevant. Indoors this can be done by continuing a carpet border in front of a service door, and painting the door and trimmings with the same paint as the walls. Different door handles can be used for cupboards and rooms that residents do not need to use. There has been awareness for some time about the need to create paths that loop around inside buildings so a person can walk without encountering physical barriers such as a locked door. By looking at a floor plan one can visually walk the corridors and room arrangements to determine if there is a connected route and what spaces it passes through. Some care buildings, especially newer ones, have been specifically designed to support this. However, unfortunately, finding such a route that also passes from indoors to outdoors is rare. In those buildings where the floor plan does appear to show a continuous loop moving through both indoor and outdoor spaces, a site visit is still essential, because buildings are not always used in the way the architect intended.

A further aspect in enabling walking is designing connections between indoor and outdoor spaces so they are in close proximity to each other. What may not seem far on paper may seem too far in reality to a person living in the home. Rooms that people regularly go to will feel closer to them than rooms they visit infrequently. The distance to the room is less of an issue than familiarity in terms of perceived distance to travel. Wayfinding is in part the result of psychological factors. Some people might find their way to a room initially but then there is the repeated challenge of finding it each time they need to go to it. But once they do get used to finding their way, it is easier not to change and go somewhere else. Unfamiliar places seem further away, even if in reality they are fewer steps away.

A physical approach also includes, where possible, designing the environment to have a secure perimeter so doors within the building can remain open. This works well in a day centre or care home with enough land to afford walking spaces on site. Fences may well be necessary but should be carefully handled so they give a strong immediate impression about the care philosophy. For example, fences can be designed to disappear from view if they are covered with shrubs and vines. Fences can also articulate domestic space, create privacy and good neighbours, enhance and open up views, as well as block light and views. The purpose of the space and how the person will enjoy it should guide the use of perimeter treatments. A person's negative or positive impressions of fences can also stem from cultural expectations.

Technological approaches

Technology provides a third approach to an overall programme of well-being for people with dementia who need to walk, and for those who love and care for them. Technology can detect and alert to a high degree of specification the movement and location of people so that a responsible person can be made aware, and steps can be taken to intervene, if the person's well-being is in jeopardy. Two types of information may be needed:

- knowing when a person goes out for a walk, and

- knowing where he is when walking.

For knowing when a person goes out for a walk, a detection system with sensors can be installed in the home. A signal is generated when a window or door opens or when a person gets out of bed. This information might appear on a computerised floor-plan of the building and a staff member would respond only if necessary. For a person living at home, if the movement (or lack of movement) detected is cause for concern, then an alert will be sent to a call centre or a neighbour, so that a designated person can respond. A modification of this system involves the person wearing a pendant or bracelet that activates a sensor.

If there is a need to know where a person is when he is walking, satellite navigation technology can locate a person in about 30 minutes by means of a tag they are wearing or a phone they are carrying. GPS-enabled mobile telephones have successfully located people to within five metres (Miskelly 2005). Database initiatives in North America, such as the Alzheimer's Society Safely Home, provide assistance when a person becomes lost. At the moment such programmes use ID bracelets but GPS is now being considered as a more efficient approach. The Alzheimer's Society UK has not followed this lead but, rather, is taking a cautionary approach to surveillance so that ethical concerns can be thoroughly explored. Wandering may be 'pottering with a purpose' requiring us to 'move beyond quick-fix practical solutions such as electronic tagging, which so often serve the needs of formal caregivers while eroding the rights of those with a cognitive impairment' and to 'develop person centred and creative ways of addressing the issue' (Cahill 2003, p.281).

Using the assessment-awareness process can lead not only to practice interventions but also to valuable insights into design, as the following story relates.

While assessing George's drive to keep moving, colleagues were:

> unable to find much of a pattern to his walks; he didn't seem to go in any particular direction, did not seem to aim for particular landmarks and did not show signs of seeking to return to previous haunts. However, we did find that if he went out for a short walk with a particular goal, such as to the local shops, he was consistently able to find his way home again. We could see from this that his mental map of his immediate vicinity was still relatively intact; as long as he stayed within these limits he was able to find his way around. (Wey 2006, p.101)

It became clear to the team that George's emotional distress was driving him beyond the limits of his immediate vicinity, and this was why he was getting lost. George had been an electrician and a keen model-maker but his life currently lacked occupation and a meaningful social role. A woodwork-based activity was initiated, and he eventually attended a day centre, which he associated with having a work-like role. Contained in his 'wandering' was:

> a striving to make sense of and act on what was going on…to curtail such actions not only does a disservice to our clients by blocking emergent tendencies within the person for growth, integration and resolution, but we would also effectively be shooting ourselves in the foot by inhibiting the processes we should be aiming to engage with as therapists, practitioners and carers. (Wey 2006, p.103)

Wayfinding, paths and surfaces

As already established, design for safe and enjoyable movement in outdoor areas involves sensitivity to the needs of older people who may be experiencing various levels of physical disability and sensory impairment – see, for example, Stoneham and Thoday (1996) for design guidance for older and disabled people in the landscape and Torrington (1996, 2004) for the design needs of older people generally. Also, design guidance is available about landscape, urban form and detailed design of outdoor environments from the IDGO (Inclusive Design for Getting Outdoors) Project by visiting www.idgo.ac.uk.

People with dementia can be disabled in their wayfinding ability, which can be impaired by reduced memory and reasoning powers. In order for a person to find his way through an unfamiliar environment, it must therefore be self-explanatory – he should be able to 'read' it. Memory impairment lessens one's ability to rely on previous knowledge, so the care environment may be repeatedly experienced as unfamiliar. An important principle in designing for people with dementia is to compensate for disability, and design has been identified as compensating by providing legibility in four different ways: visual access, cueing, spatial use and sensory stimulation (Judd, Marshall and Phippen 1998). The first two, visual access and cueing, are related and are now discussed below.

Visual access and cueing

Visual access can be achieved indoors through open-plan design that allows people to look across and observe various spaces that might normally be obscured by walls. Visual access can also be achieved by having windows along corridors looking into communal areas, so people can preview the space before they arrive at the doorway into it. Furthermore, visual access to outdoors – in particular in rooms with windows looking in more than one direction – affords people a sense of orientation both within the building and in relationship to outdoor surroundings.

Visual access can be applied in designing for nature in several ways. Primarily it is essential to ensure that visual access to usable outdoor areas is possible from indoor rooms where people spend time and which have access to the outdoor area being viewed. While outside people need to be able to see where they are in relation to the surroundings and to potential spaces they might want to visit. Visual access must, however, be balanced with the need to provide small-scale, domestic-sized places in which people can feel comfortable, which may need to be enclosed by hedging or trellises. It is also necessary while outside for people to have visual access to the way back in. So visual access can thus be viewed as a three-way street.

Cueing can aid navigation by compensating for memory loss. Indoors this can be done through colourful personalisation of a fixture such as a bedroom door or by putting a display case in a corridor filled with identifiable objects. Walls, doors and floors can also be treated with colour or texture to draw attention, for instance, to rooms like the toilet. Cueing can be accomplished outside by placing meaningful objects along paths and at decision points. A person may not remember to take the second left but may instead be prompted to turn at the yellow wheelbarrow full of lavender – see text box 'Cueing'.

Cueing

Focal points, signs and handrails aid wayfinding, and multiple cues are better than one. Robust cueing is multi-sensory and involves sound, smell and touch as well as sight. People with severe dementia were shown to thus be able to reach certain destinations in a wayfinding study by Passini and colleagues (Passini *et al.* 2000). The goal is to give simple choices and clear information about what a person can expect to find at a destination. This can be accomplished even if a destination can be arrived at from two different but easily visible routes, with one offering perhaps a richer or different sensory experience (Bennett 2006).

Spatial use, personality and stimuli

A third way in which design can provide legibility is to use spaces for specific functions so they present an identity to the person. Indoors this works if rooms are consistently used for a particular activity. People with dementia tend to avoid rooms in which the function of the room is ambiguous (Torrington 2004), perhaps because they are unclear of what they are supposed to do in it. Colour contrast can be used to reinforce difference and this and texture can be used in rooms to give them a richness a simple cream and beige decor cannot (Bennett 2006). Distinctive rooms will be more easily recognised and will aid navigation. Two lounges with different colour contrasts, furnishings and decoration (and which are perhaps used at different times of day to take advantage of changing outdoor views) will be 'read' as individual, identifiable places, helping people know where they are and what they can expect to occur there. Similarly the same results can be achieved by defining certain areas with a distinctive personality and using them consistently for identifiable activities, such as a group sitting area under the arbour.

A fourth way in which design can enhance orientation concerns an over- or under-abundance of sensory stimulation. A balance must be struck in which 'the environment is engaging without being confusing; directive without being manipulative; supporting while still promoting autonomy' (Judd *et al.* 1998, p.17).

Movement in three-dimensional space

Another aspect of 'reading' the landscape involves people's kinaesthetic sense, meaning the way they move in space. Impaired reasoning can affect physical mobility by reducing spatial awareness, including perception of three-dimensional space. For example, they may no longer understand steps leading up and down. Or they may see steps where there is in fact only a change in colour or pattern on the ground. It's therefore important to avoid giving false information when the ground is actually level and to give accurate information by the use of stepped skirtings and by installing nosings of a contrasting colour along the front of each step (Pollock 2003).

Steps in outdoor areas tend to be avoided it at all possible, depending on the particular topography of a site, leaving only slopes and ramps for building access. But in order for a landscape to be therapeutic it must also offer people a choice of challenging things to do. All people are entitled to cardiovascular health and opportunities to maintain this should not be reduced by design. Steps provide good exercise and can be provided alongside a ramp as an optional route, with a handrail on both sides. To ensure both a degree of challenge and opportunity are provided, carry out a risk assessment and then design accordingly.

Paths, slopes, materials and destinations

Paths generally need to be constructed of a consistent material and colour. However, a change in either of these can be used to give a signal to walkers that they are entering a different space. For example, a patio could have a slightly lighter colour than the space for walking into and out of it. The colour must not be too different or it is likely to be perceived as a step and therefore avoided. Also the patterns in paving of paths have been known to contribute to movement, with Utton (2007) finding that a highly visible jointing pattern can aid direction-finding and movement. The usual safety concerns also apply to paths – such as making all walking surfaces free of tripping hazards. Gravel is not a suitable surface for a path for people in a wheelchair, on a walking frame or with an unsteady gait. The surface needs to be uniformly smooth but non-slip. Pavers and concrete blocks are suitable if they do not shift and become uneven over time. For instance, avoid block pavers under large trees because the roots will tend to lift and unsettle them. Poured surfaces such as tarmac or concrete provide smooth walking surfaces. The rubberised surface used in play areas is also suitable as it minimises injury from falls. Manhole covers, if they occur in a pathway, should be recessed into the pavement and disguised with the same paving material.

Clearly it's important to consult accessibility guidelines in your locality when determining dimensions of path widths and the slope of ramps. People using a mobility aid or a wheelchair should be easily accommodated, with extra room in front of seating areas. Ramps should be introduced only as necessary with a gradient that is gradual and continuous. Paving material should be fixed and firm with surfaces such as asphalt and concrete generally being the ideal, to which colour additives can be added to reduce glare, introduce variety and distinguish between paths and edges (Bennett 2006). For a discussion of the pros and cons of different path surfacing materials, it's useful to consult Thrive information sheet 125 (Puddefoot 1996), and sheet 200 (Gould 1993) for construction process guidelines for path-laying. (Thrive is a national charity in the UK that uses gardening to change the lives of disabled people by promoting the benefits of gardening to individuals and organisations, as well as teaching techniques and practical applications. They publish a series of useful information sheets which are referred to throughout the text.)

Perhaps most importantly, paths should provide a reward for going down them. Besides actively inviting wandering and encouraging exploration, they should have structures, features and plantings that attract interest and encourage conversation and occupation. They can offer varied opportunities for enrichment, stimulation, pleasure and freedom, which many care-environment gardens fail to do, and which goes unnoticed until such qualities are missing, 'scarcely realised until denied' (Gibson 2006, p.65).

Figure 5.3 illustrates a number of aspects of the outdoor space mentioned above. This outdoor area has optional paths leading to a seating area. One has steps and the other has a slope. There are different surfaces and materials including wooden decking, concrete, pavers and grass. The choice of path will reveal a different set of experiences along the way. Importantly, the destination is understandable in terms of what is possible for the person deciding to make the effort. The visible presence of seating, a table and the raised planting beds give very clear information to people with dementia about what happens in these spaces and therefore what they are able to do if they go to them. The visible presence of raised beds also adds to the seasonal changes, as a person can see different kinds of plants growing at different times of year.

Neighbourhoods and destinations

An essential component of any neighbourhood is how well connected you feel in it to places where you want, or need, to be. Having destinations we value within easy reach increases our satisfaction with a neighbourhood. Older people most likely grew up in an environment where walking and bicycling were more commonplace than today. Research participants were found to have retained detailed knowledge of their old neighourhoods, including street names and how long it took to walk a certain route. Living close to the countryside,

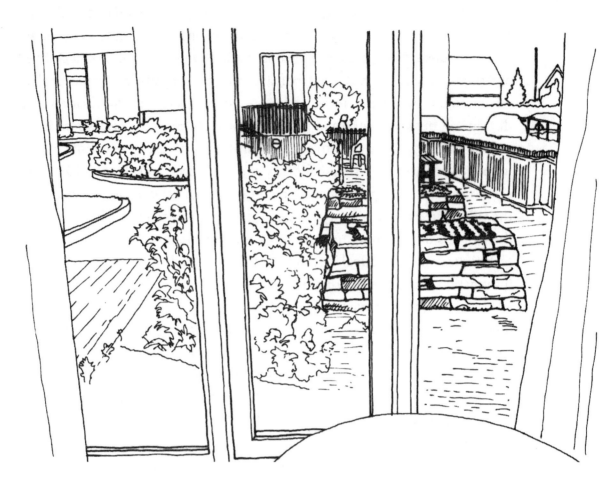

Figure 5.3 Outdoor view informs, Norway

'about ten minutes walk uphill', and being able to easily walk to it, was a valued aspect of where they lived.

Another aspect of walking is to celebrate yearly festivals. For instance in some northern communities, the Whit walks are a celebratory occasion tied to the church calendar when whole communities turn out, people take great pride in dressing in their Sunday best, children wear their new spring outfits and there is much pleasure in the social gathering.

Figure 5.4 shows maps of two different residential neighbourhoods in Yorkshire, UK and illustrates the nearness and convenience of public facilities as well as the green space and habitat areas that are within close proximity to the two care homes. Members of care staff from both of these homes regularly go out walking with residents to the shops, the post office or the pub.

In a care environment, going for a short walk outside after lunch to a special area with an excellent view and comfortable seating in the sunshine can become an activity that people look forward to. This is a regular practice in one care facility in Stockholm, Sweden, and on the walk people stop by the vegetable patch and pick flowers and baby carrots. When they reach the benches they are in a warm sunny spot, sheltered from the breeze, with a grand view of the sea as it enters the city.

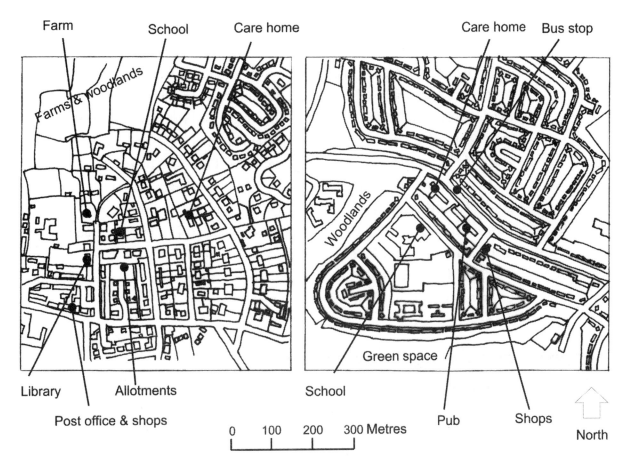

Figure 5.4 Neighbourhood walks and habitat, UK

Further south, in a day unit in the Scottish Borders in the UK, people:

feel that perhaps they want to escape from the constraints of the service. They want to have the opportunity to do what they want and when they want. Getting outside, taking in the fresh air, putting one foot in front of the other, is something they can do without being afraid of doing it wrongly. Walking off the anxiety, attempting to decrease the confusion and going down familiar streets means memories of happier times flood back, anxiety starts to decrease and they begin to feel more secure and more composed. (Wilson 2006, p.49)

'Neighbourhoods for Life' was a three-year research project culminating in 2004, carried out by Oxford Centre for Sustainable Development (part of the Department of Architecture in the School of the Built Environment at Oxford Brookes University). The project took existing literature and design guidance for the needs of older people with dementia, as well as the existing current knowledge of best practice for internal environments, and applied it to the neighbourhood level. The research aim was to explore ways in which design features in the outdoor environment affected the ability of older people with dementia to understand and navigate their local urban neighbourhoods.

Findings showed that familiarity, legibility, distinctiveness, accessibility, comfort and safety all appear to have a major influence in helping people with dementia negotiate their local neighbourhood. Small street blocks with direct, connected routes as well as distinct architectural features helped people find their way around. Services and facilities within walking distance with adequate seating, lighting, shelter, and well-maintained, smooth, level, plain paving were also helpful, especially for physically frail persons (Mitchell *et al.* 2003). The project researchers produced a checklist of recommendations and design guidance for creating dementia-friendly outdoor environments (Mitchell, Burton and Raman 2004). For example, when planning for people with dementia to take outdoor exercise and walks into local areas it is essential to consider their personal safety and well-being since their impaired reasoning powers will increase their vulnerability in areas of traffic.

Shopping and visiting the post office

A recent Swedish study found that having an extensive social network seems to act as some protection against dementia, and that people with a poor or limited social network had a 60 per cent increase in their risk of developing dementia (Fratiglioni *et al.* 2000). What this study also underscored was the importance of the local shop and post office in maintaining such a network.

Living in a care environment removes the need to provide for oneself – for example, handling one's own money – but memory loss prevents a person from actually remembering that she is no longer responsible in those ways. It is therefore common for residents to worry about having money in order to pay when they go into the dining room, or about getting to the shops, or about picking up their pension from the post office. Moving into a care environment reduces a person's routines and related purposeful walking. It also reduces the repeated, caring and knowledgeable social exchanges they had with local people and post office workers. Through a post office, a longevity of social contact with community members is established and maintained in just a few minutes of time spent regularly over the years.

Conversations both with shopkeepers and with other people in queues cover a complete range of topics, from births, holidays and hip operations, to catching up on the latest news. A sense of community is generated by smiles, handshakes, grumbling and gossip. As well as visits to the post office people might also have visited the greengrocer, the butcher and the newsagent – further opportunities to be recognised and spoken to by name. When a person speaks of a need to go shopping or to the post office this may relate to multiple losses. If a person with dementia says 'I need a loaf', she is indicating lifelong habits that may now be going unsatisfied, including social interaction and community participation. In order to partially address this need, some care homes provide a shop in which residents can use their purses and choose old-fashioned sweets, birthday cards or hair nets. On the level of neighbourhood, such needs of older people should be reflected in the design of urban regeneration schemes.

Implementation

Person with dementia

Be aware that people with dementia:

- may enjoy having a personalised physical exercise programme

- may enjoy participating in a dog-walking programme

- may be constantly walking because of multiple discomforts or types of distress

- need to walk freely to destinations of interest when and if they desire to do so.

Social environment

- Take regular walks with the person to destinations he identifies as meaningful.

- Be aware of, show concern for safety and upkeep of, and use with frequency, the nearby green spaces at an easy walking distance from the home.

- Consider taking a 'spirited walk' with people to discover their unique spirit.

- Become involved in or start a weekly walking group.

- Ensure people have identification on them and a phone number of someone who knows them and what time they are expected back – not their home address in case the person and his or her keys were to fall into the wrong hands. The person's name and phone number can be stitched into a garment or engraved onto an ID bracelet worn around the wrist like a medical alert bracelet.

- Adopt a needs-driven approach to walking by considering the effects of a range of factors on the person's ability or desire to walk (i.e. lack of privacy or sensory discomfort).

Physical environment (specific to design professionals and commissioning bodies)

- Highlight areas where a person is encouraged to go and downplay irrelevant areas.

- Create looped paths both inside the building and between its inside and outside.

- Design the property with a secure perimeter so doors can remain open within the site.

- Downplay fencing by covering it with plantings and vines.

- Design for wayfinding using visual access, multi-sensory cueing and colour.

- Maintain consistent colour and material on paths unless it is signalling a change.

- Ensure paths offer stimulation, enrichment and meaningful destinations.

- Design indoor and outdoor destinations in close proximity to each other.

Message: Design environments that enable a person with dementia to take a walk, alone and with others, to meaningful destinations, in order to derive all the benefits walking can provide.

SITTING IN THE GARDEN

A major survey on the role of private urban gardens showed the perceived value they hold for human well-being through personal enjoyment (Dunnett and Qasim 2000). The experience of sitting in a garden is enjoyable because of its effects on all of the senses. Hernandez (2007) conducted post-occupancy evaluations of outdoor spaces of two special care units of assisted living facilities for people with dementia in the USA and found sitting outdoors to be one of the most frequently recurring outdoor activities. One participant in the Edge Space Study (Chalfont 2006) mentioned memories of smelling the flowers and the trees. Her memories were also of eating food her father had grown in the garden when she was quite young.

However, whether or not this bombardment of sensory stimulation is actually of benefit to a person with dementia depends on a number of variables. Seating and shelter must be thought through and designed in order to facilitate a pleasant experience by considering in some detail the required structures and the existing micro-climates (see text box 'Visits to a garden and self-rated health'). Views into and out of the site must be treated sensitively because while there is the potential for positive social interaction with neighbours, there is also a possibly confusing intrusive experience from traffic noise, rowdy neighbours or radios. Providing a choice of seating options can also put the person with dementia in control.

Visits to a garden and self-rated health

A study by Rappe, Kivelä and Rita (2006) described the relationship between the reported frequency of visits to an outdoor green environment and self-rated health in 45 female nursing-home residents. A strong positive association was established between the reported frequency of visiting outdoors and self-rated health. The main hindrances related to outdoor visits were lack of assistance and uncomfortable weather conditions. The results suggest that it might be possible to promote the well-being of older individuals living in nursing homes by providing them with more opportunities to visit outdoor green environments. By increasing the accessibility and attractiveness of the outdoor environment, the frequency of outdoor visits might also increase, resulting in better perceived health.

Seating and shelter

When designing outdoor seating there are a number of points to consider, including the seat, backrest, arms, construction, comfort, style and materials of the seat, and its ergonomic design and location within the garden. For a good discussion of these options refer to Thrive information sheet 212 (McChesney 1995a). As mentioned earlier, seating should not conduct the cold in winter or the heat in summer. For this reason, metal furniture may be inappropriate in full sun in the summer if it becomes hot to the touch. Likewise because it conducts cold, metal furniture used in the winter needs to be placed in the sun. It is traditional to have wrought-iron Victorian benches in English gardens, as well as older gardens elsewhere. It is also popular to have stone benches, either white pre-formed concrete in the Italian classical style or natural-cut stone slab benches in contemporary gardens. Although any stone bench will conduct cold straight through a winter coat, when stone is warmed in the sun it radiates that warmth – which can be a very pleasant sensation, both to the hand and the bottom.

Since many outside areas in care homes have no seating at all, it may seem a bit indulgent discussing styles and materials of benches, particularly since plastic is so 'cheap and cheerful'! But it is important to do so because if seating is done correctly, it increases the likelihood that an area will be used, and also increases the enjoyment of people while using it. Plastic chairs and tables offer no support for people trying to steady themselves while sitting down or standing up. They also shift and slide about when kicked or bumped and a plastic table if bumped will lead to spilt drinks. Furthermore, plastic chairs will easily tip over if weight is not applied evenly to both arms of the chair at the same time, or if the chair is on a slight incline and the person shifts body weight in that direction. Nonetheless, plastic chairs rarely get too hot or too cold, don't rot or rust, will outlast many of the residents, can be hosed down, stacked and stored, are portable and can be quickly used in another part of the home, so they do have some purpose – if only for people who are steady on their feet for whom sturdy support is not necessary.

Wooden chairs will need to be painted or treated and, despite this, will eventually rot – especially quickly if they are placed in the shade where algae and moss can take hold. However, wooden chairs and benches can be heavy and sturdy, their backs and arms can be leaned against, and they don't conduct heat or cold. For these reasons wooden seating is often appropriate, especially if placed in the sun.

On the other hand, wooden tables get dirty and stain easily and require tablecloths if people are to eat or drink on them. Wood also can warp and splinter. Although wood will last longer if it is covered in winter, the sight of furniture covered with sagging plastic covers collecting puddles of wet slimy leaves is off-putting enough to make someone avoid the area entirely. Although such a view is unpleasant, seeing a bench from indoors is advisable, so a resident knows it exists, and seeing a bench sitting warmly in the sun is an attractive sight. Rocking chairs, gliders and swings can be very enjoyable, even comforting with their rhythmic movement.

The solution to the problems of outdoor seating must be dealt with on a case by case basis. A range of different styles and materials will be needed depending on the location of the seating and the time of day and time of year it can potentially be used, given the direction of the sun, the micro-climate of the location and the visibility and proximity from indoors.

Another factor to bear in mind is that furniture must not be too low or too deep, as people need to be able to get out of it easily. Its arms must protrude slightly to help people pull themselves forward and push up. All furniture outdoors needs to be periodically brushed off and wiped clean, certainly before it is used. Wooden built-in seating is sturdy, but because it is often hard and upright, it is not designed to support ageing bodies comfortably. Cushions will be needed by an older person sitting on practically any solid outdoor furniture for more than a few minutes. Cushions need to be stored somewhere nearby and periodically need to be cleaned or replaced.

Shelter from the sun while sitting in the garden can be provided by an umbrella at individual tables, by an awning that can be unfurled at the edge of the building or by a free-standing arbour or canopy over a larger area. A tree can also provide shade if it is positioned east of a morning seating area, south of a midday seating area and west of an afternoon seating area. Providing shelter is essential for people with dementia and other people on various medications who may suffer from over-exposure to sun.

Proximity of people to one another on seating is another issue to bear in mind. A shared bench does not allow for personal space but individual seats are often spaced so far apart that conversation is difficult or impossible. One good compromise to these conflicting needs is a wooden two-seater unit with a table in the middle between the two seats. There is usually a hole in the middle of such a table for an umbrella. What this configuration offers is another person within talking distance but also the possibility not to engage if preferred. Outdoor seating and shelter, because of the challenges they present the residents and the difficulty in getting the design issues right may contribute to the under-usage of outdoor areas by reducing the desire of a person with dementia to use them.

Views and neighbours

Most of us enjoy watching what is going on and an environment that affords such views will be stimulating. But it is only enjoyable if the views are controllable. The person watching needs to be in charge of initiating the view and of shutting it off when she wants to. Clearly, indoors this can be accomplished using curtains. However, outside a view must be gradually opened to the person as she is ready for it. Total exposure is uncomfortable. Fences with partial openings from different areas allow a person to choose where to sit to either open or close the potential view, both outwards and inwards. Choosing a view is also about choosing how exposed one wants to be to the outside world. If there are neighbours within the view, then the desirability of seeing them may well depend on positive or negative experiences associated with former neighbours.

One participant remembered sitting in the garden with her housemate. A man came regularly to cut the grass and trim the hedges. When asked about the garden, besides the grass she remembered trees 'up at the top' where there used to be 'a next door garden', in which a neighbour grew roses and different coloured flowers. She then recalled that if they asked him, he would give them some roses. Another participant mentioned there being a 'garden next door' with 'flowers and things'. This awareness of neighbours stayed with the participants into later life, facilitated later by the nearness of the 'garden next door', and also on the person's ability to control these views to a degree.

Routine use

If a garden or outside area is routinely used it provides more frequent benefits. Routines are comforting because they seem to give a structure to the day and this reinforces failing memory. For instance, if a person cannot remember whether or not a meal has occurred, if he knows what time it is he can make the deduction, 'Oh, well we must have already eaten if it's two o'clock'. If certain places or rooms are always used for certain meals this further aids orientation, so that if the person is in a certain room he knows it must be meal time, which then stimulates anticipation and receptivity to that activity. The outside can be used in the same way. If an afternoon drink is routinely given in the garden, then a visit to the garden may prompt a person's anticipation and perhaps increased enjoyment of that drink. Likewise, if she is sitting in the garden, she may be more receptive to drinking, because she is expecting it to occur. In this way, place and activity reinforce each other and provide some security about what is likely to occur.

Establishing routines in outdoor areas will ensure they are used regularly – or, indeed, that they are used at all. One-off visits do not establish a momentum or a flow to the day. There will be people who would enjoy a routine walk out into the garden to a warm sunny spot after a meal. Some people may turn down an offer to go outside if they feel someone is making a special effort on their behalf. But if there is a routine flow to it people may be more inclined to go along.

Visible from inside the home

The expression 'out of sight, out of mind' can be especially true in the case of outdoor areas for people with dementia. If people are asked if they would like to go outside, and they have no view of where that is, are they more likely to decline? Or does visibility from inside the home not matter? This is an area in need of further study, but from data I have collected through observations over three years in two homes, the former would seem to be the case, for some people at least. Without a clear view of the place in question, those asked often tackle the question about outdoor space creatively, as described below under 'Emotional and psychological factors'.

A further aspect about visibility within the garden itself is that this can prompt active gardening. One family carer told of her mother's usual Sunday visit to the carer's for dinner. While outside she lingered longer than usual because she became interested in pulling weeds. Being in the garden encourages people to do things – purely as a result of the enticement of nature.

Emotional and psychological factors

When asking a person about an outdoor area that he cannot at the moment see (even though he frequently visits and enjoys the place) that person may not believe he knows the area. Consequently he may come up with various reasons for not going there. There could be another place he says he prefers, which may not actually exist. He might say it is too hot or cold outside, or he is just 'not

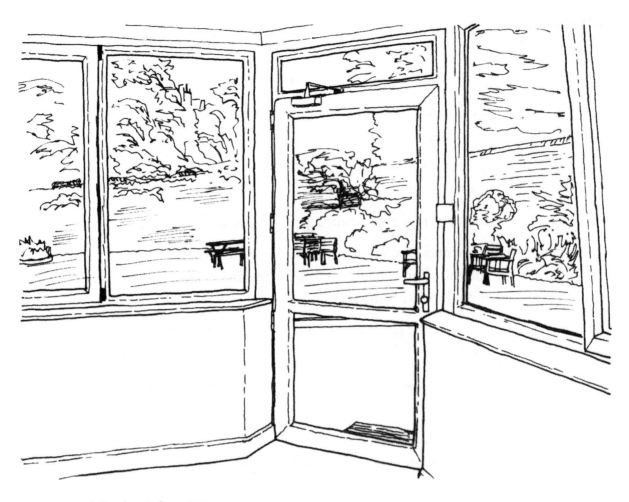

Figure 5.5 Visibility from indoors, UK

bothered'. When the reasons for not using a space in the home do not relate well to the actual places that exist, this may indicate that the person has no accurate information to base a decision on, and so may be relating the question to previously known places. One participant mentioned she liked 'to go upstairs, on top' although the home didn't have an upper level. When asked about the patio outside, to which she was a frequent visitor, another resident did not think she had ever been to it. If there seems to be emotional or psychological reasons for declining an offer to participate, it may be helpful to try to determine what exactly the person is basing a decision upon. Design can help play a role in separating fact from fiction for people who cannot rely on memory when responding to suggestions to participate. Designing outdoor spaces so they are visible from rooms of the home will enable a person to respond to reality when asked if he or she would like to go out there.

Implementation

Person with dementia

Be aware that:

- people may enjoy simply sitting in the sun, looking at trees and watching birds

- people may also enjoy interacting with friendly neighbours who they routinely see

- someone may enjoy knitting, reading or drawing outside

- a person's location must be considered in terms of view, micro-climate, furniture (for example, a table for personal items) and who might be within speaking distance

- sitting in the garden is often the first essential step towards active gardening

- pleasant sensory experiences of enjoying a place can be remembered for years

- a person may turn down an offer to go and sit in the garden because she may be thinking about another garden or space from a previous place where she spent time.

Social environment

- Neighbours can be a positive influence offering social interaction over time.

- Established neighbourhoods have potential for interaction over the fence, because older people can often be found outside tending their gardens.

- Having a friend to sit out with and share space can extend the time spent outside.

- When inviting people to go outdoors, seeing the area helps them to decide.

- Routines can facilitate the use of outdoor areas.

- Always keep a first-aid box on hand when people are outside.

- Protect a person who may be unaware that he is being over-exposed to sun.

Physical environment

- Outside areas should be visible from rooms with access to them.

- Seating
  - Use stable, sturdy furniture so people can steady themselves as they move.
  - Use seating of different materials and configurations and place it to take advantage of different micro-climates, from warm and sunny to cool and shady.
  - If using metal or stone seating (for instance for reasons of character, style or durability), ensure comfort by placing the seating in full sun during the winter. Consider using cushions to protect from heat or cold.
  - Make use of seating units that have two chairs and an integrated table in the middle.

- Plantings
  - Plan for fragrant plants through the year, remembering also fragrance from trees.
  - Trees attract birds to a garden so plant trees within earshot of seating areas.
  - An expanse of lawn highlights bird activity, making them easier to see.

Message: Make sitting in the garden a reality for people by attending to the seating, shelter, views and neighbours, routine use and visibility from inside the home.

GARDENING

Private gardens make up about three per cent of England and Wales – approximately one million acres. Over 80 per cent of houses in Britain have private gardens. These home gardens contribute to people's well-being by providing an opportunity for self-expression and offering physical and physiological benefits, as well as restorative experiences (Catanzaro and Ekanem 2004). Furthermore, domestic spaces in a home, such as the garden, have a significant influence on the scope that older people have to retain a sense of self-determination (Percival 2002). In fact, there is little doubt that home environments can have an enormous impact on the overall well-being of elderly people (Stoneham and Thoday 1996), by improving their quality of life and contributing to healthy ageing. Also, evidence suggests that 'work' in the garden has many positive benefits. However, although simply 'being' in a garden can be a source of pleasure and enjoyment, the ageing process inevitably separates one from active gardening (Bhatti 2005).

The most commonly cited reason that older people move into residential care is their growing inability to cope with their garden (Spurgeon and Simpson 2004). For older people, the inability to garden can be a form of bereavement leading to low morale (Bhatti 2006).

Why garden?

There are many psycho-social and health benefits for older people if they carry on gardening, especially being able to control their own physical space. This is important at a time in their lives when levels of control in other areas may be diminishing. Therefore, to have the opportunity to be in the garden to do something that is creative and active, that brings happiness and pleasure is crucially important to an older person's feelings of 'being at home' (Bhatti 2006, p.338).

> In a garden, one is constantly aware of and stimulated by changes in the seasons, the lifecycle of plants and insects, changing weather patterns – by all the miracles of nature. (Dennis 1994, p.xv)

Gardening also demonstrates the value of caring, patience and persistence, and produces tangible rewards.

For people with dementia, the simple pleasures of being in the garden, the physical environment, its structures and features as well as the garden plants resonate decades later in memories that come alive during conversation. These were not extraordinary places of towering aesthetic or horticultural achievement, but simple, pleasant and practical places where ordinary family life and gender roles played out. These gardens 'didn't have a lot of fancy stuff' but mainly 'vegetables and things'. Three participants in the Edge Space Study spoke of relationships with family members who were keen gardeners. Here is Edith's memory.

GC: Was there a family garden that you do remember?

Edith: A family garden that I do remember. Yes, there was one. Oh, further up the road, lower down from here, and that was me father-in-law's garden. He was a keen gardener. And that was nice, he was always out in the garden, and that was nice.

GC: What can you remember him doing?

Edith: Well mainly it was vegetables and things. He was a lovely man, a keen gardener.

GC: How did you learn about the garden?

Edith: Just by following round…like an idiot (chuckles).

GC: What did you help do?

Edith: Well, carrying a bucket or simple little things; 'bring me that bucket, Edith'. Yes, they were golden days, all gone now.

Helping father usually ended in being told teasingly to stay out of the way. Gardening was reported as being pleasant and productive with 'something nice to fetch in from outside'. In particular, roses were a favourite garden flower, remembered for being fragrant and 'sweet' smelling.

For a person with dementia to carry on gardening in a care environment or perhaps to take it up for the first time requires an environment capable of responding to specific needs. There is little evidence-based design guidance on gardens for people with dementia, although there is widespread agreement about design principles and criteria for dementia-care gardens generally (Pollock 2001). There also exists a body of work on therapeutic horticulture and some research specific to horticultural activities in dementia care. For practical guidance on design considering the literature on therapeutic gardens can be useful. In this section we will draw from these three sources to come up with a few insights for care practice. This is an interdisciplinary area in need of focused attention if care environments are to enable people with dementia to have a satisfactory gardening experience.

Social and Therapeutic Horticulture (STH) and Horticultural Therapy (HT)

As discussed in Chapter 2, STH and HT can improve the physical, mental, emotional, social and spiritual state of participants. Some reasons for this cited by participants in a study of over 800 active STH programmes in the UK included 'nature' and 'freedom', sanctuary and safety, socialising, work and employment, nurture, organic gardening and sustainability (Sempik, Aldridge and Becker 2003). When carried on outside, there are physiological benefits derived from exercise, fresh air and vitamin D from sunlight, and psychological benefits such as looking forward to something and feeling successful. Such activities are a good way to test concentration and retention, and as such can be incorporated into an interdisciplinary assessment and treatment approach.

For people with dementia, STH and HT also offer opportunities to become actively involved and to socialise with others with similar interests. Involvement promotes motion and muscle strength, and connects the person's awareness of time to a seasonal event. Projects might include: drying and working with herbs, flower pressing, transplanting, mixing soil, cutting flowers, arranging flowers, washing pots, planting bulbs, picking vegetables and planting seeds and cuttings (Hewson 2001). It also can offer chances for privacy, as people in institutional settings often lack moments of time spent alone.

Therapeutic gardens

Although all gardens have some therapeutic potential for certain people at certain times, a 'therapeutic garden' is specifically designed with the intention of achieving goals for those who use it. For this reason it is useful to refer to STH and HT when considering the design of outdoor spaces in which people with dementia can garden. Within these disciplines there is some consensus that therapeutic gardens are 'outdoor facilities for therapeutic gardening [which] reinforce and evoke a wide array of positive responses through growing, harvesting, processing, observing, and experiencing plants in their garden environment' (Kavanagh 1998, p.287). We are also told that, 'the purpose of any therapeutic garden is to maximise the number, quality and intensity of interactions with plant materials in the garden landscape' (pp.287–288). Furthermore, it is through 'active participation in the horticultural tasks of the garden or through passive appreciation of garden spaces and features' that these benefits can be recognised (p.288).

It is also recognised that there is a need to design for disability, requiring the application of universal design principles (equitable use, flexibility in use, simple, intuitive use, perceptible information, tolerance for error, appropriate and anticipated physical effort and size and space for approach and use). The seven shared traits of therapeutic gardens listed below are also relevant for people with dementia in care environments:

1.   Features are modified specifically to improve accessibility to plants and gardening techniques.

2.   Activities are scheduled and programmed.

3.   Perimeters are well-defined.

4.   There is a profusion of plant and people interactions.

5.   Conditions are comfortable and supportive.

6.   Universal design principles are used.

7.   The garden is a recognizable place.

(Kavanagh 1998, p.289)

Within this framework the garden must also remain functional, practical and safe. As when designing a horticultural therapy garden, a dementia-care environment will benefit from a thorough study of the proposed programme of activities and the existing and possible site characteristics. This needs to be done during the site-analysis phase of the design process. The goals and objectives for the use of the gardens must also be agreed upon by the design team, which includes the design professional, the home manager and members of the care staff, with input and insight from residents. Once the goals and objectives have been agreed upon then the site can be selected, inventoried and assessed for being able to meet them.

Furthermore, it's important to ensure that the garden design translates the values of the dementia-care programme into the spatial attributes on site. For instance, the layout, colour, texture, materials and surfaces for paving will have an effect and quality specific to their use by people with dementia. For a comprehensive description of the design process from which these points were drawn, see Kavanagh (1998) and also Thrive information sheet 216 (Thrive 1995).

A successful design process will result in a landscape that directly relates to the proposed activities. Dementia-care gardens stand to fail if this type of approach is not used and the gardens and their uses are left to chance, or the objective and goals are not identified. Sadly, many garden areas intended for use by people with dementia in care environments are not actually being used – a situation that will perhaps continue until their therapeutic potential is seriously recognised, and design is systematically applied to attain such outcomes.

The planting in a garden should also be specific to the needs of people with dementia. This can include sensory plants, which can increase pleasurable stimulation, prompt memories and provide cues for orientation (Kerrigan 1994). Although there has been much interest in sensory gardens for people with dementia, sadly, many of these places which were funded and installed to great fanfare now go unused, in part because they were not conceived as an integral part of the building and its routine uses. This is an issue that is addressed in other sections of this book, but here it is important to stress that the use of sensory plants in the garden can be powerfully therapeutic and should therefore be considered overall in the planting scheme of a facility, not just in a designated area. More information on this can be found in Thrive information sheets 177, 182 and 206 (which give basic general principles of garden layout, selection and use of sensory plants) as well as in numerous books on the topic of sensory gardens generally.

One particularly authoritative resource book on garden design for people with dementia has been produced by the University of Stirling and addresses the issues of the patio, paths, resting and sitting areas, enclosure, furnishings, vegetables, herbs and edible plants, trees and shrubs, plant choices, paving materials and workmanship, and aftercare. Pollock incorporates the sensory qualities of plants throughout the garden design, including tree choices, edible plants and vegetables (see Appendix 2), and seating areas with fragrant, colourful or tactile plants nearby (Pollock 2001). For more on the therapeutic value of trees and choices for therapeutic environments, see Thrive sheet 213, which addresses shade, memory prompts, visual prompts, fragrance, year-round interest, active and passive enjoyment, placement and view (McChesney 1995b).

Water is an essential aspect of all nature and is another way to provide sensory stimulation in a garden. Landscapes in care environments tend not to contain waterfalls, ponds and fountains unless they are of a very limited scale. Water features can be designed with little or no standing water to eliminate all hazard of drowning. There are many ways to design a water feature to give the sensory qualities of water, to accentuate the sound of water or to provide the visual and tactile experiences of water flowing over a surface. Although few older people today had a water feature in their own home, the pleasant and soothing effects of water in the landscape of a care environment may offer therapeutic benefit in the same way such features improve hospice gardens and cancer wards if they are properly and routinely cleaned and maintained. (It's important to obtain guidance on good practice from the Health and Safety Executive (www.hse.gov.uk) to eliminate the danger of *legionella* bacteria, which can occur in outdoor water features that emit a spray.)

Another, perhaps overlooked means of achieving a garden with therapeutic qualities is to design plantings that are culturally specific to the people using the garden. Many plants originally from overseas will thrive in the temperate climate in the UK. In fact, there are relatively few 'native' species in Britain today as much of the flora now here originated from other parts of the world and arrived here with traders, plant hunters, immigrants and invaders (Gaskell 1995). This article (also reproduced as Thrive information sheet 220) is a good introduction to multi-cultural gardening and includes useful references for further reading. When people cultivate plants from their area of ethnic origin it can remind and reconnect them to the plant's economic, religious or mythological significance, helping them grow a living connection between their homeland and the places in which they now live. Gaskell provides various resources, including a list of hardy plants suitable for cultivation in Britain, three examples of multi-cultural community gardens, some useful addresses, places to visit and further reading.

Accessibility, raised beds and greenhouses

Due to the physical changes from ageing, older people wanting to garden outside will require certain adaptations. As people's clarity of vision diminishes, so their depth perception is diminished. Bodily strength, agility and balance become compromised. The body is less able to adapt to temperature changes and a person can develop chronic health conditions. Accessibility involves making adjustments for the older person, such as enabling gardening when the temperature is the most comfortable; providing a stool and adapted and brightly coloured tools; providing large seeds to plant; water and juice to drink; ensuring they rest frequently, and wear a hat and gloves and use sunscreen. Social modifications to enable older people to garden include allowing plenty of time; arranging for them to garden with others in a safe and secure place; keeping costs low; and encouraging social and inter-generational activities in the garden. Accessibility also requires design of the physical environment to include paving and planting beds.

Any paving must meet accessibility standards concerning widths, slopes, passing spaces, turning radii, curbs and doorsteps in front of doors. Aspects of paving and surfaces specific to older people are equally relevant to people with dementia – for instance, the use of tinted concrete to reduce glare. There are also dementia-specific design criteria such as the need to diminish any visual difference between paving areas of different materials to avoid the appearance of a step. If two different materials are to be used, for instance concrete and tarmac, they should be tinted in such a way as to diminish the difference where they join. Paving should also not appear shiny or reflective because it can then be perceived as water, which a person will avoid for fear of slipping and falling.

Handrails may be required at entrances to buildings and on slopes depending on steepness, but they are also useful in other places to assist with balance and mobility. Access to lawn areas should be at the same level as the adjacent pavement, but the edges of pavement adjacent to planting areas should have raised curbs to keep wheelchairs and walking frames on the path. (For a good overview of hard surfacing for disabled and elderly people, see Thrive information sheet 125, Puddefoot 1996.) Design for wayfinding, paths and surfaces was also covered earlier in this chapter under the heading 'Wayfinding, paths and surfaces'. Another important issue of accessibility is ensuring that toilets are nearby. This is crucial for people with challenges to their physical mobility and has a bearing on their decision to visit the outdoor areas at all.

To provide a garden experience that is both flexible and diverse, both traditional and container planting situations should be provided. Traditional planting includes:

> ground-level beds and borders; slightly raised beds and borders, which
> may be encased with some stable materials as a kind of curb or edging; and
> raised beds or borders [see Figure 5.6], which can be completely supported
> by retaining walls made of a variety of materials. (Kavanagh 1998, p.299)

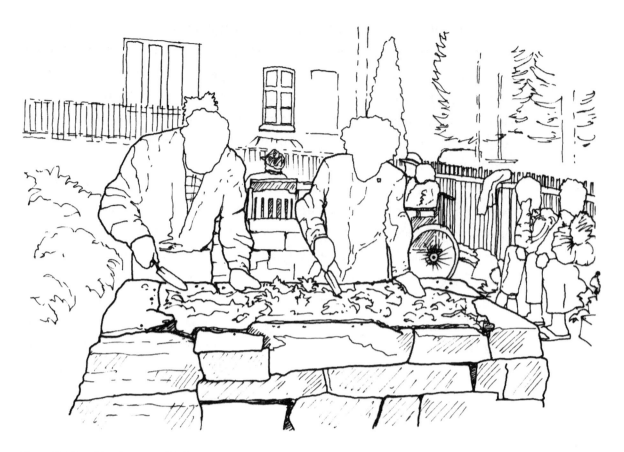

Figure 5.6 Working in a raised bed, Norway

Container planting utilises containers, window boxes, tabletop planters, hanging baskets and a variety of pots. It brings the advantage of complete control over the quality of the soil and greater flexibility about where the gardening and the growing takes place. Vertical planting (for instance, using trellises) increases the available space in the garden in which plants can actually grow. There are very specific assets and problems associated with each of these planting situations including watering, cost, soil, space availability, accessibility, comfort, climate, convenience and economy (Kavanagh 1998, pp.300–301). Help on ways to build raised beds can be found in Thrive information sheet 184.

The benefits of a greenhouse are that it creates growing and gardening space and makes it available all year round. There is also a benefit in that both day and night it can provide fragrance and moisture that stimulates the olfactory senses leading to the limbic system, the largest emotional part of the brain (Hewson 2001). A greenhouse is a project, not just a structure, and there needs to be someone on hand who is passionate about it and will keep it maintained and in use. Logistically, it should be placed in an area that includes seating, a patio area, a table and a tool shed. It should also be out of the wind and close to a door of the building that is regularly used by residents. In order to remind people with dementia that it exists it should also be visible from inside the home. Generate discussion about the greenhouse, drawing on the life history of the residents, many who will have had experiences with family members who were keen gardeners. A short walk out to see what is growing in the greenhouse can be worked into the flow of the daily routine. Family care-givers and volunteers with green fingers may also enjoy being involved with a greenhouse.

Kitchen gardening

When 106 people between the ages of 60 and 94 were surveyed about using their gardens in sheltered housing compared with previously in their own homes, they reported that:

- 80 per cent used to garden compared to 15 per cent now

- 40 per cent used to grow vegetables compared to 0 per cent now

- 55 per cent used to grow cut flowers compared to 8 per cent now

- 65 per cent used to grow cuttings compared to 10 per cent now

(Stoneham and Jones 1997, p.22, Figure 2)

What this shows is not just how much productivity has been lost through a decline in gardening activities, but also the high general rate of productive gardening in which older people were engaged when in their own homes. Perhaps the greatest impediment to kitchen gardens in care environments is that home-grown produce will not be grown if it cannot be consumed on site. Rather than be a disincentive, health and safety regulations must be challenged in areas where research or care practice indicate potential gains for residents. This should not, however, be a disincentive to growing food, as it can be taken home by family members and staff instead.

Kitchen gardens can be located conveniently near the kitchen in a sunny spot and produce a range of edible and useful plants. In addition, a small outdoor area can become transformed from an institutional landscape into a garden where a range of fruits and vegetables can be produced, including apples, pears, raspberries, blackberries, currants, cucumbers, squash, tomatoes, beans and rhubarb.

Herbs can be grown on a sunny windowsill indoors, or in a pot or raised bed outside, and then pinched off and used in cooking. Herbs can also be grown in a pot by the door so people smell and touch them when coming and going, and so that their smell can waft into the home when the windows are open. Herbs need sun and soil that dries out between watering. Choose easy-care and common herbs like mint, thyme, chives and parsley.

Sunflowers are an easy plant to grow and provide bright yellow flower heads and seeds for birds. Sunflowers were found growing in a small garden plot

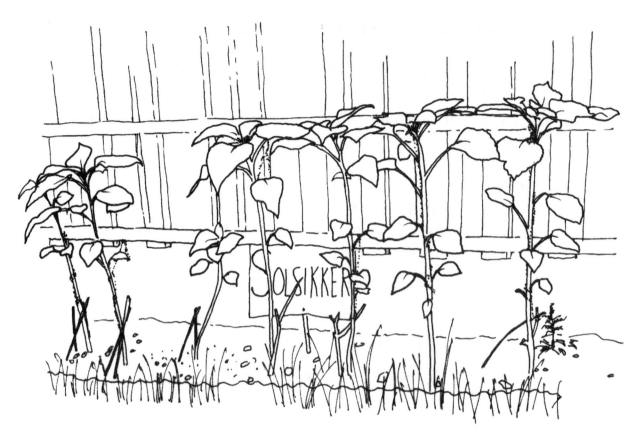

Figure 5.7 Sunflowers growing, Norway

outside one dementia care home in Norway, visible from the kitchen window, with the sign 'Solsikker' (Sunflowers) (see Figure 5.7). Notice how the young stems are staked with small sticks. They were then tied to the trellis with string. Tomatoes and cucumbers can be grown in a greenhouse, and people can be involved in checking them from time to time as they ripen, picking them, carrying them in, washing, preparing, serving and enjoying them in a meal. Fruit trees can provide apples and pears, and beans are easy to grow and can climb up an existing fence. A clump of rhubarb is virtually indestructible and can be divided every few years.

Allotments are common around the world and many older people will remember going to the allotment with their parents or gardening on one themselves. Developing an area on the care home property where families or volunteers can come to garden, and involving the residents in it, will rekindle those memories. The work and the pleasure of gardening and harvesting remain vibrant in memory for some people with dementia and opportunities to remain involved in these to any extent, even passively, are very likely to be enjoyed by them.

Implementation

Person with dementia

Remember that people with dementia:

- will have a degree of impairment and functioning level that will affect their participation in gardening activities

- may be on medication that increases sensitivity to sun and may therefore burn easily

- may not perceive the sun as being too hot and may need prompting to cover up

- may be unaware of the cold or unwilling to admit they are too cold rather than inconvenience someone to go in and get their coat or cardigan. Lack of temperature sensitivity can be disease-related, while not asking can be cultural.

Social environment

- Be aware of participants' impairments and limitations, keep an activity simple, speak clearly and strive for fun and enjoyment.

- Activities should meet the person's physical and mental capabilities and be a means of achieving optimal levels of accomplishment.

- Ensure the activity results in a meaningful outcome for the participant.

- Involve volunteers and family members.

- If outside, supply participants with hats and apply protective sun lotion.

- Always keep a first-aid box on hand to treat bites and stings promptly.

- Be aware of which plants are poisonous (see Appendix 3); keep a plant book on hand for easy identification and check labels of plants you are buying.

- If at all possible, decide that projects are going to use organic methods.

- See that tools are safely stored and regularly serviced. Use appropriate tools for the job – tools the participants are familiar with – and carry out a risk assessment.

Physical environment

- If possible, kitchen gardens should be placed very near to the kitchen.

- Install trellises, pergolas, bean poles and wires as frames for vertical plantings.

- Use adapted equipment and environments to address physical limitations.

- Ensure the area has shade protection by using umbrellas, awnings or trees.

Message: Provide opportunities and environments for people to continue to enjoy gardening or to take it up as a new hobby in order to gain some of the many benefits it is known to provide.

DOMESTIC ACTIVITIES

Much of normal domestic life involves people in experiencing elements of nature such as the sun and wind, leaves and wildlife. Putting out the laundry requires a person to be aware of a multitude of climatic conditions any time of the year and to be able to respond quickly if they change. Sweeping and raking are both vigorous healthy activities exercising the heart and lungs as well as the legs and the upper body with a range of bending, stooping and squatting. Feeding wildlife such as birds and squirrels as well as domestic animals such as chickens requires a set of mental and physical skills. Each of these domestic activities ties a person not only to the landscape but to the climate and to living nature (in the form of trees or animals), and also to the turning of the year, as well as providing exercise and movement.

Essentially, domestic life is about maintaining relationships with nature, ourselves, neighbours and our physical homes. It requires skills of stewardship and care-giving that are essential to maintaining our humanity and our sense of connection to the world. Pottering in the garden is a meaningful and enjoyable occupation that means different things to different people, as the following qoute illustrates:

GC: Do you come outside much?

Edith: Not an awful lot. I do it when I'm at home. Potter in the garden. And, uh, well I just think it's a... a pleasant thing to do. You know you can sit in the garden, you can garden, or you can potter in the garden, or go and visit somebody and enjoy being out with people, you know, it's got a lot for it, sunshine.

It seems to be a very individual and obviously satisfying pastime because pottering is not something somebody else can do for you, unlike any other garden task. Similarly domestic activities are an important component of dementia care, regardless of whether or not that person still lives in or maintains his or her own home. Pottering can include organising, tidying up, moving

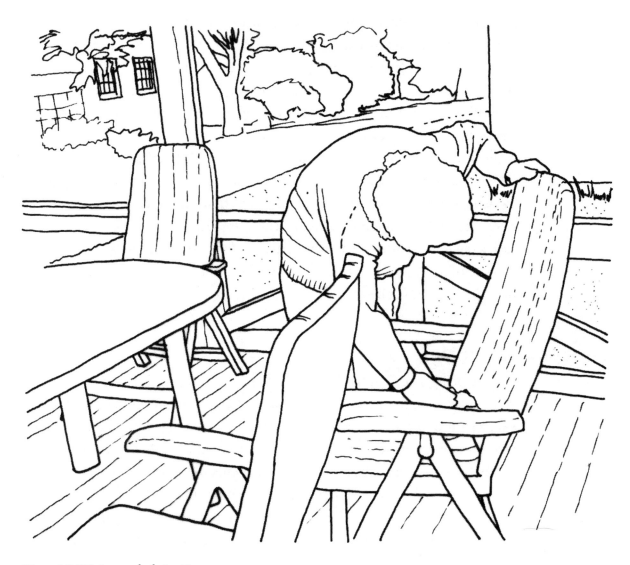

Figure 5.8 Wiping porch chairs, Norway

things about, transferring materials from one place to another and wiping or cleaning outdoor furniture (see Figure 5.8). Such acts of maintenance are essential to wholeness. Opportunities for continuity should be found so a person can continue to have these daily acts of domestic engagement with nature as part of their routine. What Figure 5.8 also shows is a close proximity to next-door neighbours in one home. During the fieldwork at this particular home, normal friendly conversation occurred between the resident in the drawing and the man living next door who came out and conversed while trimming the shrubbery. The importance of this will be taken up later, in Chapter 6, when we consider the ethics of social contact with neighbours and visibility in the community.

Hanging out the laundry

Whether or not it is a good drying day depends on how strong the wind is, whether there is sun or rain, and what are the temperature and humidity – all factors in the drying time of a load of laundry. Ascertaining such information depends on being acutely aware of the time of year and hence the rotation of the sun around the garden during that day. Being able to forecast the potential drying time for a load of laundry requires a person to look outside and gauge such things, and also to be able to react quickly if the environment changes and it starts to rain. The physical acts of carrying washing outside, reaching up and pegging a piece one at a time onto the line, spacing items so they all fit, pegging them in such a way they hang neatly and dry thoroughly, taking them down and folding them, carrying the clothes basket in (and sometimes folding and putting away the clothes line if it is portable), are all activities that require a broad range of manual and spatio-temporal skills. There are few other activities that require such a range of abilities, all of which have tended to become lost with the advent of the clothes dryer – a technology unheard of in the life experience of many older people with dementia.

Sweeping and raking

Besides being good cardiovascular exercise, sweeping and raking can provide great satisfaction from effort expended. There is a pleasure and satisfaction to a swept path or a raked lawn that is unrivalled when compared with activities where there is no obvious visual outcome for the work. There is also the opportunity to engage socially with others while outdoors, as there is often the chance for a neighbour to 'supervise' the job underway. This type of outside work also extends the season, since one can keep warm outside by moving about as opposed to sitting still. Such outdoor tasks are often tied to the changing of the seasons, such as leaves falling, or to the cycle of the week, such as sweeping the paths as part of your Saturday chores. For a person who may be losing touch with time of day, days of the week or time of the year, activities can reinforce temporal orientation. Just being outside can give the body messages about what time of year it is. There is also the basic human need to remain independent and to care for ourselves and our homes, to the extent we are able to, for as long as possible. In this sense, engaging in domestic housekeeping rituals can be therapeutic beyond the point when they are done expertly or achieved up to a certain standard.

Feeding the birds and squirrels

Watching birds come to a feeder can both occupy and entertain. Many people will have routinely made this connection to wildlife for years while living in their own homes. Every effort must be made to allow people to continue to feed and watch the birds, if that was what they used to do. Many older people have taken up bird-watching because they finally have time to do so. Squirrels are notoriously tame when food is on offer and will even destroy bird feeders to get to the seed! A squirrel can be trained to come to a certain spot and eat peanuts, which can be a delight to watch from indoors, especially in the winter. People often give names to a bird or squirrel and befriend it, training it to come at a certain time each day. These relationships can be as sustaining as that of a pet and should be given equal significance.

Bird-feeders should be placed in relationship to the windows and to seating areas, or wherever people are most likely to be able to watch birds come and go. A view of a feeder from the dining room may actually stimulate eating as well as conversation. A bird-house outside a bedroom window at a height visible from seating inside will provide hours of enjoyment. Keeping a bird-identification book, and a diary and a pen near the window will enable bird sightings to be recorded. A bird-table is not always necessary, as evidenced by one resident who fed birds from her bedroom window. However, if people inside are to be able to watch bird activity outside then a bird-table is necessary and must be placed within view and filled with seed routinely. Providing binoculars would be a bonus.

Feeding the chickens

People with dementia today who grew up in rural places might well have kept domestic animals or livestock. Gathering eggs, milking cows, feeding the chickens or shooing the geese out of the vegetable patch would have occurred routinely. These domestic caretaking rituals played a role in the maintenance of the family and tied a person to the place through physical and emotional engagement with nature in daily life. Opportunities to reawaken such practical, meaningful contact with nature through daily caretaking routines should therefore be sought. The ADARDS (Alzheimer's Disease and Related Disorders Society) Nursing Home in Tasmania cared for 31 ambulant residents and had strong connections to outdoor areas, including a chicken coop and an aviary in the garden, as well as an old blue car for polishing.

Implementation

Person with dementia

Remember that:

- the person will have once carried out, and may have enjoyed, housekeeping chores outdoors when growing up or during later life. Many older women in the north of England can still remember scrubbing the industrial soot off their front steps

- women will have been very aware of moisture and air movement as they would be the ones to decide whether or not it was a good day for drying clothes

- the person may have been raised on a farm and have stories to tell about the animals

- feeding birds and squirrels may be an especially meaningful activity.

Social environment

- Determine which domestic activities people once enjoyed (which may be gender-specific) and re-enable such activity in their current living environment.

- Allow and encourage people to participate in domestic tasks such as sweeping, raking and putting out the laundry, which involve engagement, discussion and co-ordination with natural forces such as the sun and wind.

- Ensure the person is appropriately dressed for outdoor activities, including wearing appropriate shoes.

Physical environment

- Design elements into the landscape such as a clothes-line or a postbox only if use of such things can be routinely facilitated.

- Build into the landscape (and into the care practice) elements such as a rabbit hutch or a chicken coop, so there are meaningful chores to do.

- Design an area of path specifically so that residents are able to sweep it.

- Design an area of lawn specifically so that residents are able to rake it.

- Facilitate an environment in which pottering is possible.

- Install bird-feeding stations so people can take part in feeding the wildlife.

Message: Provide opportunities and environments for people to continue their routine, meaningful, domestic activities of maintaining and caretaking around the home.

TAKING A TRIP

Chances to take a trip independently, to go to the pub or the park, to drive, to take the bus or to fly abroad are often severely curtailed for a person with dementia. There are multiple reasons for this, including a disabling physical environment and a diminished social network, the stigma of dementia within a society, as well as a general invisibility of people with dementia and therefore a lack of understanding of their design needs. This section will mention three types of trips that have been identified as pleasurable and often missing for a person – going out for lunch, day trips and going on holiday.

Going out for lunch

Going out to a pub, café or restaurant may have been something a person with dementia had previously done on a fairly routine basis. Neighbourhoods in which such social activity generally occurs usually have establishments close to where people live, in which a clientele of 'locals' can develop. In this situation it is more possible for a person to continue to walk to the pub or café once she has moved into care as she will be recognised by the staff, owner or other customers. A care home with a pub nearby can arrange to walk residents there for dinner (the noon meal in the UK). Any trip outdoors enables people to experience nature and is therefore to be encouraged. Going to lunch can be the main purpose of the trip but side trips for shopping are always popular.

A successful care service initiative for people with dementia is the 'flexible outreach' programme, which enables people with dementia to continue doing meaningful activities. One such programme facilitated a visit to the churchyard for a woman with dementia to visit her husband's grave, something she had not been able to do on her own. It is essential to help people with dementia to maintain a purposeful connection to the local area through activities such as this. If a trip out can be organised to include a meal out, a walk to the shops or a bus ride, this kind of social engagement can be maintained. For example, one daughter regularly took her father out to a pub in the country each week. The waiters soon came to know him, what he enjoyed eating and his favourite lager. Even when he had difficulty remembering their names, 'He always remembers faces,' she said.

Day trips

There are numerous places to go and things to do that are tied to seasonal changes or that involve animals, wildlife, agriculture, gardens or local natural areas such as parks, lakes and the seashore. Try to take advantage of local natural resources – for example, a visit to the local farm during lambing season or to the petting zoo will provide opportunities to enjoy watching or making physical contact with animals, as well as the social interaction with the farmer or other local people. Make sure you have investigated the accessibility features and the availability of toilets beforehand.

The garden-centre café is another popular destination surrounded by plant life. For people with a high degree of mobility, places where you can pick your own fruit offer a relaxed informal environment in the fresh air and the opportunity to eat while you pick. Such activities are fail-safe as there are no expectations to be met. The person can simply experience and enjoy the moment. Natural environments such as a strawberry field or a farm offer a wealth of stimulation with which people can engage at their own speed and under their own accord. Such environments offer constant stimulation. They are also authentic, useful, practical places with clear intentions about what happens in them and what outcomes can be expected. There is no ambiguity about why you are there and what there is to do. Social interaction is a bonus, not the main event.

Just getting out in the bus and riding around can also be stimulating and enjoyable for people, and is an experience that often stops when people move into a care home rather than just visiting it. When one person who visited a day centre for several years moved into residential care and began living in the care home rather than visiting it in the minibus, she experienced a period of confusion during which time she felt she was still coming to the day centre. Because she still had expectations of going out places and doing social activities, which was now much less common than before, she was confused and disappointed. She told another resident, 'It's a beautiful day, we could have been paddling our feet in [the river].' Her perception was understandable given her history of attendance at the day centre.

In this particular home caring staff members came in on their day off to take the residents out on trips but they identified weather as being one of the greatest impediments, as well as the availability of toilets and wheelchair facilities. Also, 'having enough staff on' is a problem as is the problem of transport. 'You can only have the bus for so long so you're limited to where you can go and what you can do', said a staff member.

A notice on the bulletin board of another home boasted a sign-up sheet for 'Our yearly trip'. But how normal is it to only go out once a year? And why are trips out not as common in residential care as they are in day care? These are important issues to consider if people are to maintain some connection to the natural world as well as to remain visible and participate in the larger community. In one dementia-care facility in Norway, photos in an album showed residents picnicking by the river, watching chickens, goats and rabbits at a family park, and riding on a dog sled in snow-covered woodlands. Cultural differences seem to play a role in what is considered acceptable treatment of people with dementia and how much effort and resources one could expect to be spent on giving such people a wonderful day out.

Going on holiday

For many families the pleasure of going on holiday with their relative after they have developed dementia is simply foregone in light of the daunting level of detail and arrangements it would require, and the fear and panic that may arise during it. Relatives have identified the difficulties and stress associated with possibly losing a person in a crowd or an unfamiliar setting. Hotels can be as daunting in their structure, lack of visual access, uniformity of corridors, poor signage and wayfinding cues as care homes. In moments of sheer panic for the family care-giver, a person with dementia may not see the problem: 'Where have you all been? I'm not lost. You'd gone. It's you that's the problem.'

The hospitality industry has some catching up to do in order to make resort destinations and the transportation between home and away far more user-friendly for people with dementia and their families. Areas such as vigorous outdoor activity holidays for people with dementia (Brooker 2001) could be promising. To experience the grandeur of nature at the ocean or in the mountains does not need words or memory, just the body and the spirit. These moments are priceless and every effort should be made to create them for people with dementia who will spend most of their remaining days living in a care environment.

Implementation

Person with dementia

Remember that people with dementia:

- may have sustained meaningful relationships through trips out, which will now need to be identified and enabled as they can no longer do such things alone

- may have taken holidays with their families, which is something they no longer do

- may forget they have been out to see something, but there will be an accumulated effect on their heart and spirit of such experiences – or lack of them.

Social environment

- Meet people's need to go out by taking them on trips away from home.

- Go with the person to the pond to feed the ducks.

- Promote the visibility of people with dementia by keeping them involved in local life.

- Find out about farms, stables or petting zoos in your area and plan trips to see them.

- Make a note of local parks, a duck pond or a fishing lake and plan a visit.

- Make efforts to include people who are less physically able on day trips.

- Always check ahead on issues of accessibility and availability of toilet facilities.

Physical environment

- Plan neighbourhoods with local amenities within walking distance.

- Design care environments in walking distance to natural areas and amenities.

- Plan holiday destinations and modes of transport that cater to the needs of people with dementia and their families.

Message: Enable a person to take trips out to lunch, into the country and out of town to experience the pleasure and fun of the authentic, practical and wonderful natural world.

Chapter 6

Ethical Issues Concerning Nature Outdoors

INTRODUCTION

Perhaps one of the most difficult ethical dilemmas in the design of dementia-care environments involves their connection to the outdoor world. Both the physical environment and the social aspects of dementia care often conspire to keep people contained and sedentary. This is due in part to the custodial nature of care necessary for vulnerable people, but is also especially acute in dementia-care practice where people's vulnerability is compounded by impaired memory and reduced learning and reasoning, high levels of stress and an acute sensitivity to the social and built environment (Marshall 1998). Containment in dementia care occurs on various levels – by encouraging people to sit down; getting people to stay together in one room such as a lounge rather than moving about; staying indoors rather than going outside and thus avoiding the local community.

ETHICAL DILEMMAS

In this chapter, as in Chapter Three, ethical issues involving nature outdoors are raised and the ethical principles applied are described. The issues raised apply to residential care or in some cases more broadly to persons still living in private homes in the community. Design solutions and insights from the research are given where possible.

Walking around in the home

A person with dementia who walks a lot is constantly being asked to sit down.

The dilemma here is one of conflicting needs – those of the person with dementia and those of the care-giver.

The person with dementia needs to be moving about for numerous reasons (as discussed in Chapter 5). Walking through the home provides an opportunity to access a variety of natural stimulation, from different levels and quality of light, to outdoor smells, to a change of view. It is now recognised that the built environment, not just people, can play a role in abuse.

> Inappropriate building design can restrict movement in and around the building, thereby limiting activity and enjoyment. Design that does not take account of a range of individual needs and wishes may create an environment which is inaccessible, hostile and which does not support recreation or physical activity. (Ferguson 2006, p.56)

Movement represents autonomy – personal independence and the capacity to make moral decisions and act on them. Walking may be one of the few autonomous activities available to the person and it is also beneficial and enjoyable exercise. Limiting a person's freedom (and the use of restraints) are serious mental-health issues for which government guidelines should be consulted (Mental Welfare Commission for Scotland 2002, 2005).

From the care-giver's perspective, a person should be discouraged from walking if (in the opinion of the care-giver) walking increases to an unacceptable level the chances of the person falling. It may also be that low staffing levels limit observation of residents who are spread out about the home. A person's physical movement may also be restricted by routine encouragement to keep together with the other residents in the lounge. The person might not like the lounge (because it's too hot, has no view, he doesn't like music being played or the television always on), or some person sitting in it. By voting with his feet, he is refusing to consent to being told where he must be.

In this context understanding a person's life-story is essential because social roles that may no longer exist are closely linked to people's self identity (Cheston and Bender 1999). Behaviour such as 'wandering' may indicate searching for those roles and making 'heroic efforts to maintain personal identity' and therefore should be reinforced rather than extinguished (Gibson 2006, p.63).

Ethical solutions here might include:

- educating care providers on research that concerns the relationship between physical exercise, for example Tai Chi, and decreased fall rate

- designing living areas with more of an open plan to reduce visual barriers between rooms and to increase the possibility of unobtrusive monitoring by care staff

- designing 'spaces for residents to be able to walk about and make their own choices as to where they want to be in the household… a looped path which is a series of events – sitting areas, corner windows, verandas, etc. so residents can safely move around according to their own moods and choices' (Utton 2007, p.134).

Attracting and feeding wildlife

A person with dementia living in a private flat has been told he cannot feed the squirrels or the birds.

The dilemma here is, again, one of conflicting needs. From the perspective of the person with dementia, supporting wildlife by putting out nuts and seeds is a routine occurrence for him, a source of joy as well as providing hours of entertainment and companionship. The person takes pride in having developed a relationship with one particular squirrel he has named and trained to come each morning to a fence-post outside his window to collect some peanuts. The perspective of the housing development is to oppose and discourage such interaction through rules against putting out food, believing this attracts rodents to the property. Since from a health and safety perspective there is also the possibility of being bitten or scratched, the owners of the property are also protecting their residents from harm. The issue is the relative importance of attracting and feeding wildlife to a person with dementia. If he forgets he is not supposed to do it, and puts out peanuts, he risks a confrontation with the owners. If he remembers he is not allowed to feed the wildlife, he might feel he has abandoned a living creature that has come to depend upon him. The squirrel at some point will stop coming to visit him. He also loses the daily contact with the outdoor environment. One design issue might also arise about the location of the feeding station. When he lived in his own home, he had a bird-feeder in the lawn. Seed that overflowed or was scattered by squirrels sprouted when it hit the ground and contributed to the lawn. In his new place, he cannot reach the lawn area so the feeding results in discarded peanut shells and bird-seed on the pavement where it may attract rodents rather than sprout and grow, or compost back into the soil.

Ethical solutions here might include:

- sweeping up the area after the squirrel has had the peanuts and left

- designing places for interaction with wildlife that are integrated into the building

- repositioning the feeder into a grassy area, or planting grass around the fence-post

- enabling the man to feed wildlife near his flat, maybe in a small pocket park

- enlightening the management with research evidence about the benefits for older people of contact with wildlife and of having meaningful, purposeful activity, in the hope that they will change their policy towards outdoor activities for residents.

Going for a walk

A person with dementia living in a care home is prevented from going for a walk — or even going outside.

Most people have an expectation that they can go outside when they want to. Some cultures consider going for a walk outside to be an integral part of each day, regardless of the weather or where the person happens to live. When taking a walk and returning is no longer possible for a person with dementia to do independently, the desire to do so can be pathologised as being 'wandering' (see Chapter 5). The fear and anxiety of care-givers about something happening to a loved one is very real and well-founded and for a person with dementia, taking a walk alone can be a risky and even life-threatening activity. It has been suggested that up to 40 per cent of people with dementia become lost at some point during their illness, and 5 per cent do so repeatedly (McShane *et al.* 1994). From the perspective of care-givers therefore, both formal and informal, going for a walk outside must be restricted to some extent. But curtailing a person's access to outdoors is an issue that raises many questions. What are the cultural values attached to keeping people with dementia indoors? What is the emotional cost to people in exchange for their physical safety? How does it alter our human relationships with people with dementia? Does it reinforce the false division between 'us' and 'them'? How does one balance a need to walk with a need to be safe while doing it? What values motivate and inform our choice between movement and freedom or safety and restraint?

Clearly, the care-giver's concerns for safety and risk avoidance must be balanced against the person's freedom and autonomy. However, to respect autonomy and to ensure beneficence, the person's needs and expressed desires must also be facilitated because, on the principle of justice, a person with dementia has the same rights as other citizens. People also have, one can argue, the right to put themselves in harm's way, if that is what they desire. One woman 'escaped' from a care home to die in the cold of night by taking very calculated actions. Her daughter believed she did much like a Native American elder would have done and 'freed herself' (Reid 2006).

Another issue here is the person's mental self-image. A lack of self-awareness of his condition can make it difficult for the person to understand why his movement is restricted. Since liberty is infringed when a person is in legal custody, a person prevented from going for a walk may be wondering, 'What have I done wrong?' This scenario can occur in both a care environment and also in a private home.

> Any restrictions on freedom of movement by others is a serious matter and
> should only be considered when an individual is at risk if out and about
> unsupervised, and when their judgment of when and where it is safe to go
> is impaired. (Lyons and Thomson 2006)

By keeping a disabled person inside are we actually disempowering that person and, if so, what design of the environment would empower that person? If we choose to curtail the person rather than redesign the environment, upon what criteria are we making that decision?

As mentioned earlier, assistive technology is increasingly being used in dementia care, including the use of certain devices to address the issue of people 'wandering'. Baldwin makes the important point that all technological devices reflect values and, furthermore, that technology not only supplies something but takes something away (Baldwin 2006). He presents the example of central heating having replaced the stove and consequently the meaning and meaningful activities associated with it. 'In terms of the design and application of technology we should take into account those focal things and practices that will be positively or adversely affected by the technology' (Baldwin 2006, p.62). Bowes, in talking about technology for people with dementia, tells us that all technological innovations occur within a social context and are stimulated by issues perceived within that context (Bowes 2007). So what is the social context for keeping a person inside? Are we protecting a vulnerable person, and if so, what aspects of the environment make the person vulnerable, and are we addressing those, as well as the person's movements?

Are we violating the human rights of a person with dementia if we use a GPS device that can locate missing people? If it can save the person from being lost, are we denying him or her access to outdoors by refusing to consent to electronic tagging? But at what cost do we restrict people's liberty and invade their privacy? When considering all the ethical issues one needs to take into account legal statutes such as the European Convention of Human Rights which preserves the right to non-degrading treatment, liberty, security and respect, in order to ensure that 'the use of wandering technology is the least restrictive intervention available and does not reduce standards of privacy for the individual' (Lyons and Thomson 2006, p.54).

> Even legal standards fail to satisfactorily address the intricate issues raised by assistive technologies in the dementia context…relegating some of society's most vulnerable to an unexamined fate, characterised by our propensity to embrace assistive technologies prior to fully investigating the ethical dilemmas that they generate. (Eltis 2005)

Ultimately, ethical solutions to this dilemma depend on values involving respect for people, rather than a choice between safety or human rights (Hughes and Louw 2002). Trying to resolve this complex dilemma will involve considering issues of privacy, surveillance, stigmatisation, safety, liberty, autonomy, mental capacity and evidence. What is in the person's best interest will 'require careful inquiry, negotiation and judgement. It is especially at this point that understanding the wandering behaviour and looking for the least restrictive ways of dealing with it will become imperative' (Hughes and Louw 2002, p.848). This approach includes:

- investigating the person's need for walking and addressing it on a daily basis

- reading available evidence and discussing it with all parties involved

- walking with the person to determine where they are trying to go. Then helping him or her learn the return route by discussing landmarks and sensory cues

- designing accessible, visible and meaningful walking routes to and from the home

- improving relationships by striving to know the person better, spending time being with him rather than doing to him (Hughes and Baldwin 2006)

- debating use of assistive technology for people with dementia including discussion of advanced directives and the greater health-care problem (Eltis 2005).

Social contact with neighbours and visibility in the community

A person with dementia sitting in a care home garden has no next-door neighbour.

> Before going to live in a care environment, one man spent a great deal of time in his garden. In spite of the course of his disease, he was able to share friendly exchanges with his neighbour over the fence. Because of the location of the care

home he has now moved into and the position of the building on the land, he now has no neighbours living near enough for him to talk to while he is in the garden. The building is positioned in the centre of the lot and the patio seating area is a small space tucked down behind the building and contained by a tall fence. The distance between the residents and the neighbouring properties is too great to make verbal or even visual contact. This design ensures the privacy (and safety from intimidation from those who would seek to do harm) of people with dementia using the patio, as they cannot be overlooked. But if people desire to make social contact they are prevented through design from doing so. The conflict here is between using outdoor space to provide social engagement and continuity for a person with dementia, and the need to ensure that the environment provides adequate care, as well as safety, security, and privacy.

This issue extends to the person's role in the community at large. In considering this it can help to look in very simple terms at social construction theory's analysis of a person's ability to maintain a sense of self. This, it argues, relies on three aspects – Self 1, 2 and 3 (Sabat 2001):

- Self 1 is personal identity

- Self 2 is mental and physical attributes and related beliefs

- Self 3 is the social personae, such as 'good neighbour' or 'loving dad', constructed during social interaction with others.

People maintain their Self 3 through routine visibility in their village or town and the public contact that visibility makes possible. Without these opportunities to communicate with people who we do not live with but who know us through our social presence, we publicly disappear. People with advanced dementia are at an even greater risk of being hidden away in nursing homes where they lose contact with, and social standing within, their community. The Wiekslag nursing home in the Netherlands cares for six people with advanced dementia. Each day one of the patients will accompany the nurse to the supermarket in a wheelchair. On these outings the person can see and be seen, thus maintaining a social presence, while selecting goods at the grocery.

SUMMARY

Four ethical dilemmas have just been examined in terms of nature outdoors:

- walking around the home

- attracting and feeding wildlife

- going for a walk

- social contact with neighbours and visibility in the community.

Because these raise issues of safety, vulnerability, risk, human rights, autonomy, physical and emotional health and well-being there are no right or wrong answers. However, simply recognising that there is a dilemma enables us to grow in our perception of the problem and to honestly own our part in it. The best solution will be one that is person-centred and considers all the viewpoints. It will enable the complexity to be recognised and the issues to be clarified. For further reading on the moral issues facing family care-givers of people with dementia, see Hughes and Baldwin (2006), who explore areas in need of ethical reflection, the concepts that care-givers use, their ethical reasoning and the ethical environment. They point out that care-givers become expert at dealing with difficult decisions, that ordinary care involves an ethical component and that reflecting on that can improve such care (Hughes and Baldwin 2006, p.9).

Finally, ethical issues must also be addressed from both the design of the social environment and the physical environment. Consider a gondola on the canals of Venice – a perfectly balanced boat that glides across the top of the water, because the design of the boat includes the weight of the gondolier. When empty, the gondola itself leans to one side. Lasting solutions can only exist at this kind of interface of human and physical need. Whatever solution is reached must also be regularly reviewed as the person's disease progresses and as the needs of all parties change.

Chapter 7

Summary

INTRODUCTION

The potential for connecting people with dementia in care environments to nature is limited only by our imagination, willingness and resolve to design nature into life. This short trip through the natural world, both indoors and outdoors, has, we hope, highlighted a number of ways in which this can be accomplished – some of which may have been new to you. Willingness to break out of traditional approaches to care practice and building design is essential if we are to resolve the general lack of nature in people's lives and the accepted level of separation between people with dementia and the natural world that is the current standard. This chapter contains four sections:

- seven key points in designing for nature in dementia care

- design for research

- design for ecological sustainability, and

- a conclusion.

DESIGN FOR NATURE IN DEMENTIA CARE: SEVEN KEY POINTS

This section seeks to provide design guidance by defining various features of nature, and drawing some action points from these.

Nature is good food

Connection to nature starts within us. Since we are what we eat it's important we consume healthy food. Skin, hair, eyes, teeth, bones, muscles, nails, heart, kidneys, digestion, weight, stamina and even our mental health are all determined in part by what we eat and drink. Healthy eating and drinking keeps people bright, alert and more able to enjoy life. A menu should offer 'living' food such as leafy greens and sprouts, fruit, nuts and whole grains.

Nature is daily life

Our lives are touched by nature when we do things such as sweeping the path, walking to the shops, baking bread or throwing bread out of the window for birds. The most normal and familiar settings and practices for dementia care are those which are the most enriched with opportunities for nature in daily life. Design for a daily routine that incorporates connection to nature into meaningful acts and movement through the building, through the day and through the community.

Nature is social and physical

Designing good care is about both people and places offering potential for engagement – from windows to walks in the country, from aquaria to outings. Walking can require both a path and a partner – both are essential ingredients of good care. According to Brooker (2006), the four key elements of person-centred care are:

- *Valuing* people with dementia and those who care for them (V) (p.12)

- treating people as *Individuals* (I) (p.12)

- looking at the world from the *Perspective* of the person with dementia (P) (p.12)

- a positive *Social* environment in which the person living with dementia can experience relative well-being (S) (p.13)

The aspect of 'Social environment' perhaps could be expanded into 'social and physical environment', to recognise the need for intentional design of people and place. Within this context nature can permeate daily life and improve services for person-centred care.

Nature is spontaneous

Design enabling environments where different energies and elements overlap. For example, create the possibility that birds might be heard in the presence of others in a comfortable setting, so that if they are heard, conversation can spontaneously erupt about this.

Nature is home

We call her Mother Earth because nature is from whence we came.

> There are deep reasons for our love affair with nature. We are creatures who evolved in an environment already green. Within our cells live memories of the role vegetation played in fostering our survival as a species. Plants reconnect that distant past, calling forth feelings of tranquility and harmony, restoring mental and physical health in a contemporary, technological world. Whether in pots, gardens, fields, or forests, living plants remind us of that ancient connection. (Lewis 1996, p.xix)

Design for nature as a starting point, not just as an end in itself, but as a doorway into ourselves.

Nature is courageous

Initiating design of care environments to afford connection to nature can take one out on a limb. So take courage and do your homework. Ask yourself, 'What is the worst that can happen?', 'What is the best that can happen?', and 'Are we making attempts to prevent harm that are of equal magnitude to the scale of harm we hope to prevent?' Design of care practice and care environments needs to lead rather than follow. The inspectorate needs evidence upon which to base requirements, so do your research. Remember, today's risk is tomorrow's standard.

Nature is everywhere

Design creatively. Dementia alters people's perception, and while we know a lot about the ways in which dementia disables an individual, we are only beginning to scrape the surface of the ways in which dementia opens a person to beauty, simplicity and the spiritual, through an uninhibited engagement with the world. The more nature we put into a person's life, the more opportunities that person will have to teach us why nature is needed and enjoyed. We can thus deepen our understanding of his or her experience, at the same time as improving design. This is illustrated in the following anecdote from a book about the spiritual dimension of care for people with dementia (Shamy 2003). Eileen Shamy, formerly a principal of a city school, had two little boys bring two frogs in a jar to her office, 'for your mother, to help her find her memory'. That afternoon:

> As I walked into the lounge of the nursing home I was aware once more of this room of sad, silent, sitting women. It always seemed to me as if they had lost themselves and each other…

…I walked quickly to my mother's chair and, kneeling down in front of her, lifted the plastic gauze top from the jar. Instantly, in a quick green arc, one frog jumped on to her hand and then sat, very still. My mother pulled herself up straight in her chair and squealed with delight, 'It's a little frog!' And then, in quiet wonder, 'A little frog.' As her eyes met mine she softly said, 'I had a frog in a jar…'

As silently and as naturally as the light rises with the sun, banishing the darkness, so life entered the room, transforming the women, so that each one was sitting up straight, eyes bright and sparkling, darting here and there, following the frogs as they jumped in wide, quick leaps across the room and from one woman's lap to another. Soon the lounge was filled with a glorious pandemonium of delighted laughter, excited exclamations, joyous relationship and two tiny, quick, green frogs.

I watched spellbound as each woman was touched to life once more. This was resurrection. Everyone was talking at once in a happy determination to share the frogs. Then, amazingly, in a lull, I heard a woman singing:

All things bright and beautiful,

All creatures great and small;

All things wise and wonderful,

The Lord God made them all.

Can we explain what happened that day? My little lads at school were absolutely right. My mother had found her memory just as they hoped she would. (Shamy 2003, pp.121–122)

DESIGN FOR RESEARCH

There is a great need for research about care environments for people with dementia that produces more understanding of such people's daily life and human needs. Much current research does not positively impact design because it fails to uncover how and why people use spaces in the way they do. Research methods such as surveys and questionnaires are merely the beginning of identifying the areas in which to look. Nonetheless, they are valuable tools for empowering people whose voices are rarely heard, and can provide quality social interaction – unfortunately still lacking in many care environments. We must treat with caution research projects that disengage with people with dementia by exclusively valuing the opinions of those around them, as this perpetuates the 'us' and 'them' culture of care.

What is lacking generally is a holistic approach to design, although there are some notable recent exceptions (see, for example, Hernandez (2007)). To understand the *how* and *why* of using space, one must spend time in that particular space, and understand 'place' as a process:

> While standing outside a care home recently wondering where we might build a greenhouse, I noticed a piece of bread and jam on the ground. The next morning it was a handful of rice crispies. Looking up, I realised it had come from a resident's window. Stepping back out of the way and watching for a moment I saw the sparrows return to their breakfast. That lady who lives upstairs is place-making every day at the building's edge. There are more birds in the garden because of her. Daily life is the action of making a place, and the edge is where most of the action occurs. Any place we investigate is merely a snapshot of a process. But by looking closely at interactions, we can better understand the energy and dynamics that drive the process of place-making and, in so doing, make better places. (Chalfont 2005b, p.342)

Humans and their environments are complex and if we want to gather findings that we can apply in design and practice, we need to observe daily life long enough to discover the relationships between people and place. Two specific suggestions follow below.

First, I would suggest that research in dementia care might benefit from the application of insights from Environment-Behaviour Studies (EBS) which seeks to understand how people and environments interact. This type of approach is more ethnographic and anthropological than the intervention studies normally used, which follow the medical model. There are relationships between people and buildings that can only be understood by observing interactions over time, as one informs the other. Both the physical spaces, and how they are used, are the result of ongoing interaction. We cannot separate what people do from where they do it. The promise of EBS lies in the three questions it asks:

1. What bio-social, psychological, and cultural characteristics of human beings…influence…which characteristics of the built environment?

2. What effects do which aspects of which environments have on which groups of people, under what circumstances…and when, why, and how?

3. Given this two-way interaction between people and environments, there must be mechanisms that link them. What are these mechanisms?

(Rapoport 2005, p.10)

Good research requires asking the right questions and having the right tools to investigate them. I am reminded of the man who lost his watch at night and was looking for it under the street lamp 'because the light's better here', not because that was where he lost it. Human beings can now probe Mars and unravel the human genome. Why, then, can we not discover what makes a person with dementia happy? I believe that the answer lies in tools. We must develop better tools and methods. The prevailing concept of measuring something like 'exiting attempts' (when a person tries to leave the situation) is concerning for at least two reasons:

- First, what *can* be measured *will* be measured.

- Second, in our hunger for evidence-based design we may be tempted to use such data, not only for the basis of design decisions, but also for judging a person's quality of life. This is so easy to do, and yet it is probably inaccurate. Design based on such research will indeed alter behaviour, but good behaviour is no evidence that a person is well-loved. If design becomes the handmaiden of behavioural control, we may be accepting well-behaved over well-loved.

The second suggestion is a cyclical model for improving dementia-care environments that includes and connects research, dissemination and design. Research needs to be systematic, transparent and routinely carried out (rather than sporadically as a reaction to a successful funding bid). Findings should not only be made available through dissemination, but fed back through design and practice innovations in a constant feedback loop of teaching and learning. In this way knowledge will be transferred to improve the environments, and the practice partners who facilitated the research in the first place will benefit in the long run. Also, ongoing efforts should be made to systematically investigate and scrutinise both the need for and the results of policy and regulatory decisions, so that policy and regulation are well-informed, evidence-based and critically evaluated. A radical approach might look like this:

RADICAL – Research And Design Innovation for Care, Architecture and Landscape:

1. Government and privately funded research and design in care and nursing homes

2. A network of care facilities designated as research and design facilities

3. Each public, private, voluntary and local authority provider has one RADICAL home

4. A research and design office located on the care home site

5. Care homes including several services, from dementia care to learning difficulties

6. Research being multi-disciplinary and provided through a local college or university

7. Students on research or design courses are funded to carry out work in care homes

8. Researchers, designers and practitioners working jointly on research and design proposals

9. Minimal cross-training between the three groups to improve collaboration and problem-solving

10. Research and design addressing the social, physical and ecological environment

11. A home being commissioned and/or re-registered as a RADICAL home

12. Inspection criteria being purposefully written to foster the ethos of a RADICAL home

13. Residents and care-givers legally consenting to a life with increased risk and opportunity

14. Research governance and RADICAL home inspection criteria being achieved jointly

15. Design being on all scales, from biotech and materials to interiors and neighbourhoods

16. Innovation, creativity and sustainability of water and energy being a high priority

17. Findings from the research done in each home being made widely available

18. Comparative findings being published yearly to routinely inform government policy

19. Work being linked with organisations of research, care, support and design

20. Such a programme, once set up in the UK, being replicated and expanded globally.

DESIGN FOR ECOLOGICAL SUSTAINABILITY

Current architectural knowledge now means we can produce buildings that are energy-efficient, recycle water, are carbon-neutral and produce electricity. As global warming has become a major threat to the continuity of life on Earth as we know it, and as the energy costs of running a home are second only to staffing costs, steps should now be taken with the care sector to reduce its environmental 'footprint' and to move towards ecological sustainability. In the UK, the Government is projected to spend £45 billion on the Building Schools for the Future Programme, which will rebuild or renew every secondary school in England over a 10–15 year period. This provides a golden opportunity to transfer this knowledge to the other end of the life-cycle.

The needs of people with dementia and older people actually sit happily alongside environmental sustainability. For instance, bringing daylight into buildings offers many benefits but also contributes passive solar heating which reduces fuel costs. Greywater recycling can be performed through a reed bed filtration system that creates habitat for fish and wildlife, reduces the extent of mowed areas and reduces the water and sewer bill. Adding a fontain or flow form to such a system provides the further benefit of a water feature. Likewise, modern efficient buildings can recover 'waste' heat and use it rather than release it into the atmosphere. Buildings that are situated to create warm micro-climates in the exterior edge spaces will draw people into the outdoor areas. Conservatories, atria, covered porches and sunrooms generate heat from solar gain. This heat provides thermal comfort to people using these spaces but also can be drawn into the home. Methane gas can be reclaimed from decomposition of waste material and used for heating. Beyond their installation costs, wind and water turbines and solar panels generate free energy, and surplus energy can be sold off at a profit. There is no reason why buildings for older people cannot be ecologically sustainable and efficient, since there seems to be no apparent shortage of power that can be generated – except perhaps, one might fear, political will-power.

CONCLUSION

Attempts to date to keep people safe and secure have ensured that people's experiences tend to be limited quite narrowly by the environments in which they live, with a lack of integration between indoors and outside, a poverty of natural light and fresh air, and a profusion of outdoor places that are off-limits for multiple reasons. Given the evidence we now have about therapeutic benefits of nature, we can now create care environments that support the person with dementia on a three-legged stool of research, design and care practice if the various professions and disciplines are willing to engage with each other.

When reflecting on ethical issues, it is clear that the individual must be at the centre of decisions likely to limit the amount and quality of nature in his or her daily life – especially where these decisions concern benefits that can be derived, including that individual's potential to gain in pleasure, enjoyment and well-being. But I am uneasy about recommending that we ensure nature in the lives of people with dementia simply because it is a benefit. Those of us living without dementia (for the moment) partake daily in the natural world without needing proof that we are entitled to it, or that we benefit in any way at all. The reason for writing this book was to demonstrate the benefits of nature, and to inspire care practitioners to think about their practice in a new way – a way that will result in an improved quality of life for people with dementia. But I want to end by stating that I don't believe nature to be a benefit: nature is a human right. To live without access to it is to live dislocated from our most primitive and essential humanity.

Designing therapeutic environments for people with dementia has no strictly architectural solutions. It is not realistic to hope that the design of gardens and outdoor areas alone will adequately address the complex needs of those we intend to use them. Where solutions lie is in relationships between professions, such as nurses and domestic workers, architects and landscape architects, those writing the regulations and those implementing them, those caring and those being cared for; relationships between people with dementia and people without. Whether we are designing a porch or planning someone's day, design is not something that can be imposed, but is something that becomes manifest. Along the edges where difference meets, design is not built, but grown. And therein lies the potential for beauty.

Glossary

Aromatherapy stream – an electric device that disperses the aromatherapy oil by cool air vaporization.

Atrium – a sky-lit central area of a building, usually with a glass roof, often containing plants.

Base oil – an odourless vegetable oil used to dilute essential oil before applying to the skin; also called carrier oil.

Bright light treatment – the use of bright light to treat disorders such as seasonal affective disorder (SAD), depression and sleep disturbance.

Carrier – often a vegetable oil, but it can be a base cream, lotion, gel or shampoo, which is used to dilute pure essential oils for aromatherapy.

Chair-rise time – the time it takes a person in a seated position to rise from a chair into a standing position.

Circadian pacemaker – the part of the brain that modulates our desire and ability to fall asleep at different times of day; malfunctioning may underlie sleep disorders.

Contra-indications – conditions that suggest a particular therapy would be unsuitable. Skin disorders and varicose veins are contra-indications for aromatherapy.

Diffusers – devices or products from candles to electric heaters used for dispersing essential oils so their aroma fills the room.

Dispersant – in aromatherapy, a non-alcoholic agent or surfactant that is used to distribute or dissolve essential oils evenly onto the surface of water.

Essential oils – the essence extracted from flowers, plants, herbs, leaves, fruits, woods and gums by steam distillation or other methods of extraction.

(the) Ethics of care – a theory that emphasises the importance of relationships, rather than justice, when deciding the right thing.

Exiting behaviour – when a person tries to leave a situation.

Greywater recycling – capturing domestic waste water from baths, showers and washbasins for purifying and reuse to save on use of potable water.

Headhouse – a building attached to a greenhouse for everything but growing (boiler, offices, lunchroom, generator, restrooms, water storage, order assembly, potting up, etc.)

High-intensity light – full-spectrum bulbs producing bright light (10,000 lux) in similar colour composition to outdoor light.

Incident dementia – 'incident' is used as opposed to prevalent. No participants in a study of incident dementia will have dementia at the start of the study, but a percentage will develop it (the incidence rate) while others will not. A factor such as exercise can then be associated with a reduced risk for developing dementia.

Infusion – a remedy prepared by soaking plant material in vegetable oil or water.

Intervention studies – intended to improve the condition of an individual or user group by evaluating the impact of a change, such as building modification or staff training.

Light carts – portable trolleys for growing small plants with fluorescent lights, shelves and zipped up plastic covers to retain moisture.

Neat form – the undiluted form of essential oils in aromatherapy.

Personalist ethics – starts with and addresses ethics in terms of individuals, their personality, personal expression and behaviour.

Snoezelen Room – a controlled multi-sensory environment designed initially for therapeutic treatment of people with mental disabilities by exposing them to a soothing and stimulating environment.

Surfactant – a surface-active agent that reduces the surface tension of two liquids. Used in aromatherapy, a surfactant acts as a dispersant between oil and water.

Synergy – the effect of two or more agents working together to produce an effect that is greater than the sum of the parts.

Time-series design – a research design in which subjects are tested at different times during the course of a long-term study.

Walkabout – 'Walkabout is an Australian pidgin (or perhaps quasi-pidgin) term referring to the belief that Australian Aborigines "go walkabout" at the age of thirteen in the wilderness for six months as a rite of passage. They then trace the path of the ceremonial ancestors of the tribe, following the exact route that those ancestors took, and imitating, in a fashion, their heroic deeds. In the UK, a walkabout is a name for organised group meetings in which members of the British Royal Family walk past assembled crowds of onlookers, meeting and chatting with various members of the public.' Definition from http:/en.wikipedia.org/wiki/Walkabout.

Aromatherapy definitions are from
http://www.quinessence.com/glossary_of_terms.htm.
(accessed 31 August 2007).

Appendix 1 The Prosentia Hypothesis

THE PROSENTIA HYPOTHESIS:
IF a person interacts with nature and another person,
they are able to maintain a sense of self.

The PROSENTIA HYPOTHESIS specific to dementia:
IF a person with dementia has a sensory connection to nature in supportive relationship
with another person, THEN interaction within this triangular dynamic can help the
person to maintain a sense of self (and may contribute to their positive personhood).
(Gilleard, 1984; Kitwood and Bredin, 1992; Sabat and Harré, 1992)

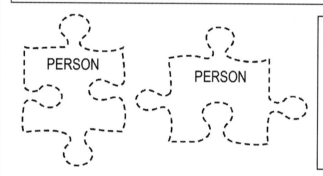

Mechanisms

SENSORY STIMULATION and
COMMUNICATION

Outcome

MANIFESTATIONS OF SELF

Proposed Model of NATURE-BASED INTERACTION facilitating SELFHOOD
(and providing the potential to contribute to POSITIVE PERSONHOOD)

Two Mechanisms

A – SENSORY
STIMULATION through
CONNECTION TO
NATURE

B – COMMUNICATION
within a supportive
RELATIONSHIP
with another PERSON

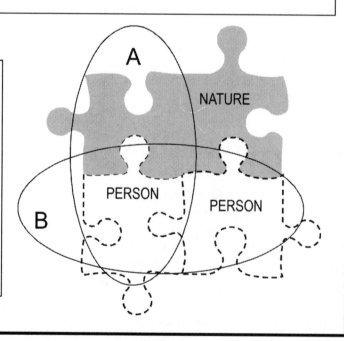

(Chalfont 2006, p.269)

Appendix 2 Edible Plants

SAFETY WITH EDIBLE PLANTS

If you intend people to be able to eat plants you will need to ensure the following:

- Avoid contaminants to the soil beds.

- Use organic cultivation methods (no fertiliser, pesticides or herbicides on the plants or in the area).

- Check before allowing someone to eat something that it is edible.

- Watch out for allergic reactions.

- Wash the plant thoroughly.

DISCLAIMER

All persons respond differently to plants and some people might have allergic reactions to them. If a plant is listed here as edible, that does not necessarily mean that it is safe for everyone to eat. Always carry out a risk assessment for individuals who may come in contact with plants, whether indoors or outdoors, edible or not. Such an assessment would need to consider what plants were available and what the likelihood is that a person would try to eat them. Persons at risk of eating plants would need to go outside accompanied by a care-giver or family member. While our aim in this book is to offer guidance on improving care, ultimate responsibility for the well-being of people with dementia belongs to their care-givers.

HERBS AND VEGETABLES

Chives, parsley, basil, fennel, licorice mint (Anise hyssop), pineapple sage, dill, cilantro, endive, escarole, scented geranium, kale, Swiss chard and thyme

FLOWERS

Nasturtium, sunflower, day lily, pearl lupin, sweet violet, borage, calendula, English daisy, pansy, rose, squash, flowers of onion, chive and garlic, flowers of guava, chrysanthemum and fuschia

VEGETABLES

Lettuce, leek, garlic, onion, shallot, squash, carrot, sorrel, potato, snow peas, garden peas, broccoli, kale, cauliflower, gourds and cucumber

SOFT FRUITS

Raspberries, strawberries, currants, blueberries, blackcurrants, blackberries and grapes

PERENNIALS

Anise hyssop (*agastache foeniculum*) and amaranthus

SHRUBS

Marshmallow (*Althaea officinalis*), Amelanchier varieties, Siberian Pea Tree (*Caragana arborescens*), Chinese, Japanese and Korean plum yews (*Cephalotaxus*), Eleagnus varieties and musk mallow (*Malva*)

TREES

Japanese dogwood (*Cornus kousa*), Ginko biloba, sassafras, service tree (*Sorbus domestica*) and lime (*Tilia*)

NUT TREES

Edible chestnut, hazel and filbert (*Corylus*), hog peanut and ground nut

FRUIT TREES

Plum, persimmon, apple, pear, mulberry, cherry, damson and peach

For some excellent ideas on incorporating edible plants into a sensory, interesting and attractive landscape visit www.gardenguides.com/Tipsand Techniques/edible.htm.

Appendix 3 Poisonous plants

All or parts of the following plants are poisonous if eaten or will cause skin irritation. Care should be taken if they already exist in gardens which a person with dementia may visit unescorted. If a person is at risk of eating plants, and potentially harmful plants are to be planted in the garden, 'site them where they cannot be easily reached' (Pollock 2001, p.29).

LATIN NAME	COMMON NAME (UK)
Aconitum napellus	monkshood
Arum italicum arum	arum lily
Atropa bella-donna	deadly nightshade
Brugmansia	angel's trumpet, tree *datura*
Colchicum	autumn crocus
Convallaria majalis	lily of the valley
Daphne mezereum	daphne
Dictamnus albus	burning bush
Dieffenbachia	dumb cane, leopard lily
Digitalis purpurea	foxglove
Euphorbia	spurge
Fremontodendron	Fremontia
Gloriosa superba	glory lily
Hedera helix	ivy
Helleborus	hellebore, Lenten rose
Heracleum mantegazzianum	giant hogweed
Laburnum anagyroides	laburnum, golden rain
Lantana camara	lantana
Nerium oleander	oleander

Phytolacca	poke-weed, poke-root
Primula obconica	poison primula
Prunus laurocerasus	cherry laurel
Ricinus communis	castor oil plant
Ruta graveolens	rue
Solanum dulcamara	woody nightshade
Taxus baccata	yew
Veratrum	false helleborine

See also Thrive information sheet 202 for a more concise list.

Appendix 4

CHECKLIST FOR CONNECTION TO NATURE IN A RESIDENTIAL CARE HOME

As discussed throughout this book, having a connection to nature is not only beneficial but is often an important part of day-to-day life for people living in their own home. Maintaining a connection to nature can be more difficult for the same person when living in a care home, unless the environment has been specifically designed to enable people to remain involved in nature. Below is a short checklist that can be used to determine the potential for connection to nature that a care home can offer. This list can help an older person, a person with dementia or a family care-giver to make an informed choice when looking for a care home. It can also be used to assist care providers to improve services, or designers to improve environments since some issues can only be addressed by a combined effort by those who commission, design, build, regulate, fund, run and work in care homes.

Name of care home _____ Date _____

Address _____

What is the weather like today? _____

VIEWS AND FRESH AIR

In order to answer each question sit in a chair in the lounge (L) and in the dining room (DR), and answer yes or no.

L / DR

___ / ___ Does the view contain trees, plants and sky?

___ / ___ Does the view contain people, traffic and real-life activities?

___ / ___ Can you see an outdoor seating area?

___ / ___ Are there trees close to the windows (to see birds and blossoms)?

___ / ___ Are there windows on more than one wall?

___ / ___ Are there any windows open at the moment?

___ / ___ Can you smell or feel fresh air in the room?

A NEARBY OUTSIDE AREA TO USE AND ENJOY

(Answer yes or no to each question.)

_____ Is there a door from the lounge or dining room to an outside seating area?

_____ Is there level access (no steps) to an outside seating area?

_____ Is the door unlocked and easy to open?

_____ Are residents using the outside area right now (or does it look like they do)?

_____ Is there outdoor furniture such as tables, chairs or benches available for residents to use?

_____ Is the furniture sturdy, clean and well-maintained?

_____ Are there any umbrellas or awnings for sun protection?

_____ Is there sporting equipment such as bowls, shuffleboard or croquet?

_____ Is there play equipment such as a swing, slide, climbing frame or ball hoop?

_____ Are there hanging baskets or planters with plants growing in them right now?

_____ Are there trees, shrubs, bulbs or plants that are visible from the seats?

_____ Is there a greenhouse, a potting bench or tool shed visible from the seats?

NATURE INDOORS

_____ Are there any live or artificial plants or flowers indoors?

_____ Do the live plants indoors seem healthy and watered?

ANIMALS AND PETS

_____ Are there any pets around (for example, dog, cat, birds, rabbit, an aquarium)?

_____ Do animals or pets regularly come to visit? (Ask the residents or staff.)

HORTICULTURAL THERAPY OR THERAPEUTIC HORTICULTURE

_____ Does an Occupational or Horticultural Therapist do nature-related activities?

Copyright © www.chalfontdesign.com 2007

References

Airhart, D.L. and Airhart, K.M. (1989) 'Inside Space and Adaptive Gardening: Design, Techniques and Tools.' In S.P. Simson and M.C. Straus (eds) *Horticulture as Therapy: Principles and Practice.* New York: Haworth Press.

Allan, K. (1994) *Wandering.* Stirling: Dementia Services Development Centre.

Alzheimer's Society (2000) *Walking About or 'Wandering'.* London: Alzheimer's Society.

Ancoli-Israel, S. and Kripke, D.F. (1989) 'Now I lay me down to sleep: the problem of sleep fragmentation in elderly and demented residents of nursing homes.' *Bulletin of Clinical Neuroscience 54*, 127–132.

ASTRID (2000) *A Guide to Using Technology within Dementia Care.* London: Hawker Publications.

Baillon, S., van Diepen, E. and Prettyman, R. (2002) 'Multi-sensory therapy in psychiatric care.' *Advances in Psychiatric Treatment 8*, 6, 444–450.

Baldwin, C. (2006) 'Reflections on Ethics, Dementia and Technology.' In J. Woolham (ed.) *Assistive Technology in Dementia Care: Developing the Role of Technology in the Care and Rehabilitation of People with Dementia – Current Trends and Perspectives.* London: Hawker Publications.

Baldwin, C., Hughes, J.C., Hope, T., Jacoby, R. and Ziebland, S. (2002) 'Ethics and dementia: Mapping the literature by bibliometric analysis.' *International Journal of Geriatric Psychiatry 18*, 41–54.

Ballard, C.G., O'Brien, J.T., Reichelt, K. and Perry, E.K. (2002) 'Aromatherapy as a safe and effective treatment for the management of agitation in severe dementia: The results of a double-blind, placebo-controlled trial with Melissa.' *Journal of Clinical Psychiatry 63*, 7, 553–558.

Bastone, A.C. and Filho, W.J. (2004) 'Effect of an exercise program on functional performance of institutionalized elderly.' *Journal of Rehabilitation Research and Development 41*, 5, 659–668.

Bennett, K. (2006) 'Designing for Walking: Creating Rich Environments.' In M. Marshall and K. Allan (eds) *Dementia: Walking not Wandering. Fresh Approaches to Understanding and Practice.* London: Hawker Publications.

Bhatti, M. (2005) *Healthy pleasures: Homes and gardens in later life.* Paper presented at the Royal Geographical Society and IBG Conference, London.

Bhatti, M. (2006) '"When I'm in the garden I can create my own paradise": Homes and gardens in later life.' *Sociological Review 54*, 2, 318–341.

Bond, J. and Corner, L. (2001) 'Researching dementia: Are there unique methodological challenges for health services research?' *Ageing and Society 21*, 1, 95–116.

Bowes, A. (2007) 'Evaluating Technology for Dementia Care.' In A. Innes and L. McCabe (eds) *Evaluation in Dementia Care*. London: Jessica Kingsley Publishers.

Brawley, E.C. (2006) *Design Innovations for Ageing and Alzheimer's*. New York: Wiley.

Brooker, D. (2001) 'Enriching lives: Evaluation of the ExtraCare activity challenge.' *Journal of Dementia Care 9*, 3, 33–37.

Brooker, D. (2006) *Person-Centred Dementia Care: Making Services Better*. London: Jessica Kingsley Publishers.

Bruce, E. (2000) 'Looking after well-being – A tool for evaluation.' *Journal of Dementia Care 8*, 6, 25–27.

Cahill, S. (2003) 'Technologies may be enabling.' *British Medical Journal 326*, 281.

Calkins, M.P. (2005) 'Learning from doing: Conducting a SAGE post-occupancy evaluation.' *Alzheimer's Care Quarterly 6*, 4, 357–365.

Campbell, S.S., Kripke, D.F., Gillin, J.C. and Hrubovcak, J.C. (1988) 'Exposure to light in healthy subjects and Alzheimer's patients.' *Physiology and Behavior 42*, 141–144.

Catanzaro, C. and Ekanem, E. (2004) *Home gardeners value stress reduction and interaction with nature*. Paper presented at the XXVI International Horticultural Congress: Expanding Roles for Horticulture in Improving Human Well-Being and Life Quality, Toronto.

Centre for Accessible Environments (1998) *The Design of Residential Care and Nursing Homes for the Elderly*. London: Centre for Accessible Environments.

Chalfont, G.E. (2005a) 'Reconnecting with nature.' *Journal of Dementia Care 13*, 2, 35.

Chalfont, G.E. (2005b) 'Creating enabling outdoor environments for residents.' *Nursing and Residential Care 7*, 454–457.

Chalfont, G.E. (2006) *Connection to Nature at the Building Edge: Towards a Therapeutic Architecture for Dementia Care Environments*. PhD thesis. University of Sheffield, Sheffield UK.

Chalfont, G.E. (2007) 'Wholistic Design in Dementia Care: Connection to Nature with PLANET.' *Journal of Housing for the Elderly 21*, 1/2, 151–175.

Chalfont, G.E. and Rodiek, S. (2005) 'Building Edge: An ecological approach to research and design of environments for people with dementia.' *Alzheimer's Care Quarterly, Special Issue – Environmental Innovations in Care 6*, 4, 341–348.

Cheston, R. and Bender, M. (1999) *Understanding Dementia: The Man with the Worried Eyes*. London: Jessica Kingsley Publishers.

Christie, J. (2007) 'Ethics, Evaluation and Dementia.' In A. Innes and L. McCabe (eds) *Evaluation in Dementia Care*. London: Jessica Kingsley Publishers.

Chung, J.C., Lai, C.K., Chung, P.M. and French, H.P. (2002) 'Snoezelen for Dementia (Cochrane Review).' *The Cochrane Database of Systematic Reviews 2002 4*, DOI: 10.1002/14651858.CD003152.

Churchill, M., Safoui, J., McCabe, B.W. and Baun, M.M. (1999) 'Using a therapy dog to alleviate the agitation and desocialization of people with Alzheimer's disease.' *Journal of Psychosocial Nursing 37*, 4, 16–22.

Cohen, U. and Day, K. (1993) *Contemporary Environments for People with Dementia*. Baltimore: Johns Hopkins University Press.

Cotman, C.W. and Berchtold, N.C. (2002) 'Exercise: A behavioral intervention to enhance brain health and plasticity.' *Trends in Neuroscience 25*, 6, 295–301.

Cott, C.A., Dawson, P., Sidani, S. and Wells, D. (2002) 'The effects of a walking/talking program on communication, ambulation, and functional status in residents with Alzheimer disease.' *Alzheimer Disease and Associated Disorders 16*, 2, 81–87.

Crawley, H. (2006) 'Food, Eating and Walking.' In M. Marshall and K. Allan (eds) *Dementia: Walking not Wandering. Fresh Approaches to Understanding and Practice.* London: Hawker Publications.

Dennis, L. (1994) *Garden for Life: Horticulture for People with Special Needs.* Saskatchewan: University Extension Press, Extension Division, University of Saskatchewan.

Department of Health (2002) *Care Homes for Older People: National Minimum Standards and Care Homes Regulations.* London: HMSO.

Dunnett, N. and Qasim, M. (2000) 'Perceived benefits to human well-being of urban gardens.' *Hort Technology 10*, 1, 40–52.

Edwards, N. and Beck, A. (2004) 'Animal-assisted therapy and nutrition in Alzheimer's disease.' *Western Journal of Nursing Research 24*, 6, 697–712.

Eltis, K. (2005) 'Society's most vulnerable under surveillance: The ethics of tagging and tracking dementia patients with GPS technology: A comparative view.' Oxford U Comparative L Forum 1 at http://ouclf.iuscomp.org, text after note 143.

Ferguson, A. (2006) 'At Risk of Abuse.' In M. Marshall and K. Allan (eds) *Dementia: Walking not wandering: Fresh approaches to understanding and practice.* London: Hawker Publications.

Fjeld, T., Veiersted, B., Sandvik, L., Riise, G. and Levy, F. (1998) 'The effect of indoor foliage plants on health and discomfort symptoms among office workers.' *Indoor and Built Environments 7*, 204–209.

Forbes, D., Morgan, D.G., Bangma, J., Peacock, S., Pelletier, N. and Adamson, J. (2004) 'Light therapy for managing sleep, behaviour, and mood disturbances in dementia (Cochrane Review).' *The Cochrane Database of Systematic Reviews 2004 2*, DOI: 10.1002/14651858.CD003946.pub2.

Fratiglioni, L., Wang, H.-X., Ericsson, K., Maytan, M. and Winblad, B. (2000) 'Influence of social network on occurrence of dementia: A community-based longitudinal study.' *The Lancet 355*, 9212, 1315–1319.

Gaskell, J. (1995) 'Multi-cultural gardening.' *Growth Point 220* (Winter).

Gibson, F. (2006) 'Lifestyle Factors Influencing Present Behaviour.' In M. Marshall and K. Allan (eds) *Dementia: Walking not Wandering. Fresh Approaches to Understanding and Practice.* London: Hawker Publications.

Gibson, S.A. (1996) 'Horticulture as a therapeutic medium.' *British Journal of Therapy and Rehabilitation 3*, 4.

Gilleard, C.J. (1984) *Living with Dementia.* London: Croom Helm.

Gordon, N. (2005) 'Unexpected development of artistic talents.' *Postgraduate Medical Journal 81*, 753–755.

Gould, J. (1993) 'Path laying explained.' *Growth Point 200* (Autumn).

Grant, C. and Wineman, J. (2007) 'The garden-use model – An environmental tool for increasing the use of outdoor space by residents with dementia in long-term care facilities.' *Journal of Housing for the Elderly 21*, 1/2, 87–113.

Growth Point (1999) 'Your future starts here: Practitioners determine the way ahead.' *Growth Point 79*, 4–5.

Hernandez, R.O. (2007) 'Effects of therapeutic gardens in special care units for people with dementia: Two case studies.' *Journal of Housing for the Elderly 21*, 1/2, 115–150..

Hewson, M.L. (2001) *Using horticultural therapy to improve quality of life for people with Alzheimer's disease.* Designs for Dementia: Integrating Systems of Care Conference, Toronto Colony Hotel. Available at www.alzheimersresearchexchange.ca/PDF/Horticulture Therapy.pdf (accessed 5 September 2007)

Holmberg, S.K. (1997) 'Evaluation of a clinical intervention for wanderers on a geriatric nursing unit.' *Archives of Psychiatric Nursing 11*, 1, 21–28.

Holmes, C., Hopkins, V., Hensford, C., MacLaughlin, V., Wilkinson, D. and Rosenvinge, H. (2002) 'Lavender oil as a treatment for agitated behaviour in severe dementia: A placebo controlled study.' *International Journal of Geriatric Psychiatry 17*, 4, 305–308.

Hopman-Rock, M., Staats, P., Tak, E. and Droes, R. (1999) 'The effects of a psychomotor activation programme for use in groups of cognitively impaired people in homes for the elderly.' *International Journal of Geriatric Psychiatry 14*, 633–642.

Hudson, R. (2006) 'Spirited Walking.' In M. Marshall and K. Allan (eds) *Dementia: Walking not Wandering. Fresh Approaches to Understanding and Practice.* London: Hawker Publications.

Hughes, J.C. and Baldwin, C. (2006) *Ethical Issues in Dementia Care: Making Difficult Decisions.* London: Jessica Kingsley Publishers.

Hughes, J.C., Hope, T., Savulescu, J. and Ziebland, S. (2002) 'Carers, ethics and dementia: A survey and review of the literature.' *International Journal of Geriatric Psychiatry 17*, 35–40.

Hughes, J.C. and Louw, S.J. (2002) 'Electronic tagging of people with dementia who wander: Ethical considerations are possibly more important than practical benefits.' *British Medical Journal 325*, 847–848.

Jarrott, S.E. and Gigliotti, C. (2004) *From the garden to the table: Evaluation of a dementia-specific HT program.* Paper presented at the XXVI International Horticultural Congress: Expanding Roles for Horticulture in Improving Human Well-Being and Life Quality, Toronto.

Jarrott, S.E., Kwack, H.R. and Relf, D. (2002) 'An observational assessment of a dementia-specific horticultural therapy program.' *Hort Technology 12*, 3.

Judd, S., Marshall, M. and Phippen, P. (1998) *Design for Dementia.* London: Journal of Dementia Care/Hawker Publications.

Kang, J.H., Ascherio, A. and Grodstein, F. (2005) 'Fruit and vegetable consumption and cognitive decline in ageing women.' *Annals of Neurology 57*, 5, 713–720.

Kaplan, S. (1995) 'The restorative benefits of nature: Toward an integrative framework.' *Journal of Environmental Psychology [Special Issue: Green Psychology] 15*, 3, 169–182.

Kavanagh, J. (1998) 'Outdoor Space and Adaptive Gardening: Design, Techniques, and Tools.' In S.P. Simson and M.C. Straus (eds) *Horticulture as Therapy: Principles and Practice.* New York: Haworth Press.

Kerrigan, J. (1994) *Gardening With the Elderly: Fact Sheet.* Retrieved 19 November 2006 from http://ohioline.osu.edu/hyg-fact/1000/1642.html

Kitwood, T. (1997) *Dementia Reconsidered: The Person Comes First.* Buckingham: Open University Press.

Kitwood, T. and Bredin, K. (1992) 'A new approach to the evaluation of dementia care.' *Journal of Advances in Health and Nursing Care 5*, 41–60.

Kryger, M.H., Roth, T. and Carskadon, M. (1989) 'Circadian Rhythms in Humans: An Overview.' In M.H. Kryger, T. Roth and W.C. Dement (eds) *Principles and Practice of Sleep Medicine*, 2nd edn. Philadelphia: W.B. Saunders.

Lai, C. and Arthur, D. (2003) 'Wandering.' In R. Hudson (ed.) *Dementia Nursing: A Guide to Good Practice*. Melbourne: Ausmed Publications.

Larson, E.B., Wang, L., Bowen, J.D., McCormick, W.C. *et al.* (2006) 'Exercise is associated with reduced risk for incident dementia among persons 65 years of age and older.' *Annals of Internal Medicine 144*, 2, 73–81.

Lewis, C.A. (1996) *Green Nature/Human Nature: The Meaning of Plants in Our Lives*. Urbana and Chicago: University of Illinois Press.

Lyons, D. and Thomson, A. (2006) 'Rights, Risk and Restraint: Guidance for Good Practice.' In M. Marshall and K. Allan (eds) *Dementia: Walking not Wandering. Fresh Approaches to Understanding and Practice*. London: Hawker Publications.

Manning, W. (2006) 'Medical Aspects of Walking.' In M. Marshall and K. Allan (eds) *Dementia: Walking not Wandering. Fresh Approaches to Understanding and Practice*. London: Hawker Publications.

Marshall, M. (1998) 'Therapeutic Buildings for People with Dementia.' In S. Judd, M. Marshall and P. Phippen (eds) *Design for Dementia*. London: Journal of Dementia Care.

Marshall, M. and Allan, K. (eds) (2006) *Dementia: Walking not Wandering. Fresh Approaches to Understanding and Practice*. London: Hawker Publications.

McCabe, B.W., Baun, M., Speich, D. and Agrawal, S. (2002) 'Resident dog in the Alzheimer's special care unit.' *Western Journal of Nursing Research 24*, 6, 684–696.

McChesney, J. (1995a) 'Are you sitting comfortably?' *Growth Point 212* (Summer).

McChesney, J. (1995b) 'Trees for therapy.' *Growth Point 213* (Summer).

McColgan, G. (2006) 'Walking with Dogs: An Alternative Therapy.' In M. Marshall and K. Allan (eds) *Dementia: Walking not Wandering. Fresh Approaches to Understanding and Practice*. London: Hawker Publications.

McKillop, J. (2006) 'Walking: A Slog or a Pleasure?' In M. Marshall and K. Allan (eds) *Dementia: Walking not Wandering. Fresh Approaches to Understanding and Practice*. London: Hawker Publications.

McShane, R., Hope, T. and Wilkinson, J. (1994) 'Tracking patients who wander: Ethics and technology.' *The Lancet 343*, 1274.

Mental Welfare Commission for Scotland (2002) *Rights, Risks and Limits to Freedom*. Edinburgh: Mental Welfare Commission for Scotland.

Mental Welfare Commission for Scotland (2005) *Safe to Wander? Principles and Guidance on Good Practice in Caring for Residents with Dementia and Related Disorders Where Consideration is Being Given to the Use of Wandering Technologies in Care Homes and Hospitals*. Edinburgh: Mental Welfare Commission for Scotland.

Miskelly, F. (2005) 'Electronic tracking of patients with dementia and wandering using mobile phone technology.' *Age and Ageing 34*, 5, 497–499.

Mitchell, L., Burton, E. and Raman, S. (2004) *Neighbourhoods for Life: Designing Dementia-Friendly Outdoor Neighbourhoods (Findings Leaflet)*. Oxford: Oxford Brookes University.

Mitchell, L., Burton, E., Raman, S., Blackman, T., Jenks, M. and Williams, K. (2003) 'Making the outside world dementia-friendly: Design issues and considerations.' *Environment and Planning B: Planning and Design 30*, 605–632.

Namazi, K., Gwinnup, P. and Zadorozny, C. (1994) 'A low intensity exercise/movement program for patients with Alzheimer's disease: The TEMP-AD Protocol.' *Journal of Aging and Physical Activity 2*, 80–92.

Oddy, R. (2006) 'Physical Activity and Exercise.' In M. Marshall and K. Allan (eds) *Dementia: Walking not Wandering. Fresh Approaches to Understanding and Practice.* London: Hawker Publications.

ODPM (1999) *The Building Regulations Access and Facilities for Disabled People Approved Document M.* London: The Stationery Office.

Passini, R., Pigot, H., Rainville, C. and Tetreault, M.-H. (2000) 'Wayfinding in a nursing home for advanced dementia of the Alzheimer's type.' *Environment and Behavior 32*, 5, 684–710.

Percival, J. (2002) 'Domestic spaces: Uses and meanings in the daily lives of older people.' *Ageing and Society 22*, 6, 729–749.

Pollock, A. (2001) *Designing Gardens for People with Dementia.* Stirling: Dementia Services Development Centre.

Pollock, R. (2003) *Designing Interiors for People with Dementia.* Stirling: Dementia Services Development Centre.

Puddefoot, R. (1996) 'Hard outdoor surfacing.' *Growth Point 215* (Autumn).

Rapoport, A. (2005) *Culture, Architecture and Design.* Chicago: Locke Science Publishing Co.

Rappe, E., Kivelä, S. and Rita, H. (2006) 'Visiting outdoor green environments positively impacts self-rated health among older people in long-term care.' *Hort Technology 16*, 1.

Rappe, E. and Lindén, L. (2004) *Plants in health-care environments: Experiences of the nursing personnel in homes for people with dementia.* Paper presented at the XXVI International Horticultural Congress: Expanding Roles for Horticulture in Improving Human Well-Being and Life Quality, Toronto.

Rappe, E. and Topo, P. (2007) 'Contact with outdoors greenery can support competence among people with dementia.' *Journal of Housing for the Elderly 21*, 3/4, 217–236.

Reid, M. (2006) 'It was My Mother's Choice to Die, and No One is to Blame.' In M. Marshall and K. Allan (eds) *Dementia: Walking not Wandering. Fresh Approaches to Understanding and Practice.* London: Hawker Publications.

Remington, R. (2002) 'Calming music and hand massage with agitated elderly.' *Nursing Research 51*, 5, 317–323.

Rigby, W. (1995) *Natural Therapies for Older People.* London: Hawker Publications.

Robertson, I.H. (2000) 'Compensations for brain deficits: "Every cloud..."' *British Journal of Psychiatry 176*, 412–413.

Robinson, L., Hutchings, D., Corner, L., Beyer, F., Dickinson, H., Vanoli, A. *et al.* (2006) 'A systematic literature review of the effectiveness of non-pharmacological interventions to prevent wandering in dementia and evaluation of the ethical implications and acceptability of their use.' *Health Technology Assessment 10*, 26.

Robson, D.G., Nicholson, A.-M. and Barker, N. (1997) *Homes for the Third Age: A Design Guide for Extra-Care Sheltered Housing.* London: E & F.N. Spon.

Sabat, S.R. (2001) *The Experience of Alzheimer's Disease: Life Through a Tangled Veil.* Oxford: Blackwell.

Sabat, S.R., and Harre, R. (1992) 'The construction and deconstruction of self in Alzheimer's Disease.' *Ageing and Society 12*, 443–461.

Savides, T.J., Messin, S. and Senger, C. (1986) 'Natural light exposure of young adults.' *Physiology and Behavior 38*, 571–574.

Schotsmans, P. (1999) 'Personalism in medical ethics.' *Ethical Perspectives 6*, 1, 10–20.

Sempik, J., Aldridge, J. and Becker, S. (2003) *Social and Therapeutic Horticulture: Evidence and Messages from Research.* Loughborough: Loughborough University (in association with Thrive).

Shamy, E. (2003) *A Guide to the Spiritual Dimension of Care for People with Alzheimer's Disease and Related Dementia.* London: Jessica Kingsley Publishers.

Sloane, P.D., Noell-Waggoner, E., Hickman, S., Mitchell, C.M. *et al.* (2005) 'Implementing a lighting intervention in public areas of long-term care facilities: lessons learned.' *Alzheimer's Care Quarterly – Special Issue on Environmental Innovations in Care 6*, 4, 280–293.

Smallwood, J., Brown, R., Coulter, F., Irvine, E. and Copland, C. (2001) 'Aromatherapy and behaviour disturbances in dementia: A randomized controlled trial.' *International Journal of Geriatric Psychiatry 16*, 10, 1010–1013.

Spurgeon, T. and Simpson, B. (2004) *Carry-On Gardening: An International Resource for Older and Disabled Gardeners.* Paper presented at the XXVI International Horticultural Congress: Expanding Roles for Horticulture in Improving Human Well-being and Life Quality, Toronto.

Stokes, G. (2006) 'We Walk, We Wander.' In M. Marshall and K. Allan (eds) *Dementia: Walking not Wandering. Fresh Approaches to Understanding and Practice.* London: Hawker Publications.

Stoneham, J. and Jones, R. (1997) 'Residential Landscapes: Their Contribution to the Quality of Older People's Lives.' In S.E. Wells (ed.) *Horticultural Therapy and the Older Adult Population.* New York: Haworth.

Stoneham, J. and Thoday, P. (1996) *Landscape Design for Elderly and Disabled People.* London: Garden Art Press.

Tappen, R.M., Roach, K., Applegate, E.B. and Stowell, P. (2000) 'Effect of a combined walking and conversation intervention on functional mobility of nursing home residents with Alzheimer disease.' *Alzheimer Disease and Associated Disorders 14*, 4, 196–201.

Thrive (1995) 'Managing design processes.' *Growth Point 216* (Autumn).

Torrington, J. (1996) *Care Homes for Older People: A Briefing and Design Guide.* London: Chapman and Hall.

Torrington, J. (2004) *Upgrading Buildings for Older People.* London: RIBA Enterprises.

Torrington, J.M. and Tregenza, P.R. (2007) 'Lighting for people with dementia.' *Lighting Research and Technology 39*, 1, 81–97.

Tronto, S.C. (1998) 'An ethic of care.' *Generations 22*, 3, 15–20.

Tyrell, J. (2007) 'Evaluating the Experience of People with Dementia in Decision-making in Health and Social care.' In A. Innes and L. McCabe (eds) *Evaluation in Dementia Care.* London: Jessica Kingsley Publishers.

Utton, D. (2007) *Designing Homes for People with Dementia.* London: Journal of Dementia Care.

Volicer, L., Harper, D.G., Manning, B.C., Goldstein, R. and Satlin, A. (2001) 'Sundowning and circadian rhythms in Alzheimer's disease.' *American Journal of Psychiatry 158*, 5, 704–711.

Watson, N.M., Wells, T.J. and Cox, C. (1998) 'Rocking chair therapy for dementia patients: Its effect on psychosocial well-being and balance.' *American Journal of Alzheimer's Disease and Other Dementias 13*, 296–308.

Weinstein, L.B. (1998) 'The Eden Alternative: A new paradigm for nursing homes.' *Activities, Adaptation and Aging 22*, 4, 1–8.

Wey, S. (2006) 'George: Thinking with His Feet.' In M. Marshall and K. Allan (eds) *Dementia: Walking not Wandering. Fresh Approaches to Understanding and Practice.* London: Hawker Publications.

Whall, A.L., Black, M.E., Grah, C.J., Yankou, D. J. *et al.* (1997) 'The effect of natural environments upon agitation and aggression in late-stage dementia patients.' *American Journal of Alzheimer's Disease and Other Dementias 12*, 216–220.

Wilson, P. (2006) '"Walking the Walk" in the Day Unit.' In M. Marshall and K. Allan (eds) *Dementia: Walking not Wandering. Fresh Approaches to Understanding and Practice.* London: Hawker Publications.

Zeisel, J. and Tyson, M. (1999) 'Alzheimer's Treatment Gardens.' In C. Cooper Marcus and M. Barnes (eds) *Healing Gardent: Therapeutic Benefits and Design Recommendations.* New York: John Wiley.

Further Resources

Further information on each of the following topics can be found on the websites listed below.

Activities	www.napa-activities.net
Aromatherapy	www.aromatherapycouncil.co.uk; www.aromatherapyuk.net
Communication	www.dementiapositive.co.uk
Design	www.chalfontdesign.com; www.idgo.ac.uk
Flowering mixes	www.pictorialmeadows.co.uk
Green roofs	www.livingroofs.org
Healthy living	www.healthyliving.gov.uk
Horticultural Therapy Social and Therapeutic Horticulture	www.thrive.org.uk; www.ahta.org
Pets as Therapy (PAT Dogs)	www.petsastherapy.org
Walking	www.wanderingnetwork.co.uk

Subject Index

Author Index